Psychiatry and Philosophy

Psychiatry and Philosophy

By Erwin W. Straus
Maurice Natanson
and Henri Ey

Edited by
Maurice Natanson

Springer-Verlag
New York Inc. 1969

Erwin W. Straus, M. D.
Research Consultant
VA-Hospital
Clinical Professor of Psychiatry
University of Kentucky
Medical Center
Lexington, Kentucky/USA

Maurice Natanson
Professor of Philosophy
University of California
Santa Cruz, California/USA

Dr. Henri Ey
Médecin-Chef
Hôpital Psychiatrique
Bonneval/France

The Contributions are taken from
"Psychiatrie der Gegenwart, Band I/2",
published by Springer-Verlag, Berlin,
Göttingen, Heidelberg
Translation of Contribution 1 from the
German by Dr. Erling Eng,
Lexington, Kentucky/USA
Translation of Contribution 3 from
the French by Stephen C. Kennedy,
Lexington, Kentucky/USA

Preface

The three essays reprinted in this book were first published in 1963 as individual chapters of a psychiatric treatise entitled *Psychiatrie der Gegenwart* (Psychiatry of the Present Day). The editors, W. H. GRUHLE (Bonn), R. JUNG (Freiburg/Br.), W. MAYER-GROSS (Birmingham, England), M. MÜLLER (Bern, Switzerland), had not planned an encyclopedic presentation; they did not intend to present a "handbook" which would be as complete as possible in details and bibliographic reference. Their intention was to "raze the walls" separating Continental and Anglo-Saxon psychiatries and to offer a synopsis of developments in psychiatry during the last decades on an international basis. The editors requested, therefore, cooperation of scholars from many foreign countries, large and small, on both sides of the Atlantic. A section entitled "Borderlands of Psychiatry", in which MARGARET MEAD (New York) discusses the relation of "Psychiatry and Ethnology", HANS HEIMAN (Bern), the relation of "Religion und Psychiatrie", and ROBERT VOLMER (Paris), "Art et Psychiatrie", is a good illustration of the trilingual character of the whole work.

Two of the editors, GRUHLE and MAYER-GROSS, died before the publication had been completed. In a kind of posthumous eulogy, Professor JUNG and Professor MÜLLER praised the initiative and accomplishments of MAYER-GROSS, "who during the last five years of his life had given a great deal of his time to this work. He had set his mind on a synthesis of German and Anglo-Saxon psychiatry. Through his world-wide contacts with scholars from all countries he was in a position to gain a collaboration of many authors and to give a fresh impetus to their own contributions. Thanks to his manifold talents, his critical evaluation, his sense for the practical and the actual, he was in a position not only to mediate between somatic and psychological research but also to re-establish a liaison between the divergent attitudes of English, American, and European psychiatries. Thus he was predestined as editor of a present-day psychiatry on an international basis."

By far the greatest part of the whole work — three volumes out of five — is dedicated to the exploration of the foundations of psychiatry

(*Grundlagen-Forschung*). Its last, or rather its final section, entitled "General Conception and Basic Philosophical Problems", contained, besides the contributions of HENRI EY, MAURICE NATANSON, and ERWIN W. STRAUS, an essay by JÜRG ZUTT, entitled "Verstehende Anthropologie", and ROLAND KUHN's "Daseins-Analyse". Alas, the task of providing adequate translations for these tractates presented difficulties which could not be overcome. Whereas the volumes *Existence* (edited by MAY, ANGEL, and ELLENBERGER) and *Being-in-the-World* (translated and introduced by JACOB NEEDLEMAN) have provided the English-reading audience with texts and commentaries to BINSWANGER's "Daseins-analysis", ZUTT's treatise deals with the still unfinished task of re-inspecting the foundations of psychiatry. Philosophical anthropology, notwithstanding its profound respect for the awesome accomplishments of science and technology, refuses to worship science in blind submission like a goddess. Instead, mindful of the fact that science is a human creation, philosophical anthropology raises the question of what enables man, a midget in the vast realm of the universe, to observe, describe, measure, and finally, to dominate the world to which he belongs.

It is improbable that neuroanatomy, neurophysiology, behaviorism, or any of the so-called basic sciences could answer this question. For all of them simply take for granted the possibility of observing, describing, measuring, and predicting. Neurophysiology especially is confronted with a real dilemma, since in every neurophysiological study at least two brains are involved: one brain as object of observation and another brain as an organ serving the observer in his studies. Usually the claim is made that the structure and function of the one observed must also account for the working of the other in spite of the fact that a brain under observation might be replaced by a heart or a kidney, while the observing brain does not yield its position. Yet no brain has ever known itself. Nor did any observer, be he a CAJAL, a SHERRINGTON, a CUSHING, ever have the slightest direct knowledge of his own brain in the way each of them was familiar with his hands, his feet, his tongue. With all their scientific wisdom, they were concerned with brains of other men or animals, not so seldom treated as if they represented an *encéphale isolé*. But in theory the tables are turned. There the expectation is that the microscopic or even molecular structure of the "mental apparatus" will eventually explain the behavior of living men and beasts.

When GRIESINGER, more than one hundred years ago, established the pathology and theory of mental diseases ("insanity") as a special branch of medicine, he raised the question, "What organ must necessarily and invariably be diseased where there is madness?" and answered: "Physiological and pathological facts show us that this organ can only be the brain. We therefore in every case of mental disease recognize a morbid action of that organ." (GRIESINGER's statement has usually been quoted with the condensed formula: "Mental diseases are brain diseases.") In a later passage GRIESINGER repeated this statement; yet in spite of this firm position in nosology, his philosophical attitude was that of an agnostic rather than a dogmatic materialist. In any case, GRIESINGER's theoretical stance is that of the observer who seeks to correlate mental states with neuro-physiological counterparts in the brain. Alterations in the former are to be explained by changes in the latter. GRIESINGER's analysis of the emotions is an interesting illustration of the essentially mechanistic, sensationistic, and associationistic philosophy which underlies his conception of mental disease. The emotions are thought of as physical balances of a sort in which changes in the composure of the individual are really shifts in the balance system. Thus, "the emotions are much more lively when, through a sudden change occurring within the consciousness, the masses of ideas belonging to the I fall into violent oscillation, and the I thereby suffers an abrupt or restless change". To interpret anger "as an acceleration of aspects" of the nervous system is, whatever else may be involved, to assume that anger is "in" the body in the same sense in which the brain is in the cranium. Or if some of the attributes of anger are not "in" the body, they are often treated as epiphenomena by those who still orient themselves along the axis of GRIESINGER's thought. What is presupposed in both the nineteenth and twentieth century versions of mechanism is an epistemological separation of mind and body, a sundering of self and world which was one of the more dubious gifts bequeathed us by Descartes. That legacy requires some comment.

In philosophical jargon, it is common to speak of the "external world", but not too often is the question asked, "External to *what*"? As with many other commonly repeated terms, "external" is simply taken for granted by both speaker and listener, writer and reader. The speaker and the writer are "in" the world, in the sense of having physical placement at the podium or at the desk in this or that portion of space. The individual is surrounded by things and related to fellow men. He participates in the events which make up our experience of the world. In Cartesian terms, the split between the two substances — mind and matter, most simply — means that the individual faces the problem of coming to know events which are outside of him. Classically, what develops as a philosophical response to the gap between self and world is a theory of the sensations which is then given the responsibility for linking the otherwise separate spheres. Thus the senses become the intermediaries between "inside" and "outside". The question, however, is not whether the senses serve their function reasonably well in this machine model of consciousness, but rather whether the model itself is adequate for comprehending and illuminating man's modes of being in the world. One of the most productive features of the

phenomenology of EDMUND HUSSERL and his followers has been the articulation of a theory of consciousness which provides a major methodological
alternative to the Cartesian portrayal of human reality (what HUSSERL
owes to Descartes in other respects is, of course, clear to any reader of
the *Cartesian Meditations*). It is at this point that the authors of the
essays which comprise this volume find a common philosophical point of
departure for the study of man.

In different ways, the three authors are agreed that the Cartesian
dualism is a metaphysical stumbling block for the erection of a satisfactory
theory of human being and human action. Phenomenology is translated
and adapted by each of them in somewhat different ways, but they agree
in interpreting consciousness as an irreducibly *intentional* structure. It is
the essence of all acts of consciousness (all thinking, willing, imagining,
judging — all perceiving, in the broadest sense) that some object is intended
by the acts in question. Thus, all thinking, for the phenomenologist, is
always thinking *of* something, all imagining is directional in nature,
positing something imagined. The "objective" status of the intended object
is not at issue. The hallucinating patient sees something, whether or not
that something is "real" for his fellow men. Further, by attending to the
directionality of consciousness, the phenomenologist is able to offer a
variegated and intensively detailed set of descriptions of the phenomena,
i. e., that which is intended by consciousness. Finally, the intentional
structure of consciousness is integral; it avoids splitting up phenomena into
either the "subjective" and the "objective", the "internal" and the "external", or the "real" and the "illusory". The full scope of conscious life is
brought into view and given legitimation. And with this conception of the
primacy of consciousness comes a new emphasis on the eminent position
of the immediacy of the world of daily life, the *Lebenswelt* within which
each individual intends and interprets the cosmos. It is within the everyday
world that the individual first comes to recognize the signs of disease,
and it is within the confines of his naive immediacy that he comes to
grasp the meaning and status of what is deemed normal. The "norm" of
the normal is defined by the decisive force of the life-world each man is
born into and bears throughout his existence. We receive no formal
initiation into the normal; we do come to learn, however, that the inversion,
pathology, and destruction of the normal is a possibility of daily life.
A phenomenology of the life-world is an inescapable task for any philosophically oriented psychiatry which seeks to elucidate the fundamental
conditions of mental pathology. With that suggestion, we come to a resting
point, if not a conclusion, in these prefatory remarks, for the relationship
between philosophy and psychiatry is a thematic concern in the essays
which follow. That relationship deserves a final word.

Philosophy and psychiatry are bound to each other. At the level of theory, any attempt to progress in a discipline succeeds fully only when the conceptual framework of the leading ideas of that theory has received proper clarification. The vocabulary and syntax of science must be attended to if the propositions it formulates are to be understood. Obviously, there are theoretical advances in the history of science whose full significance becomes clear only after much work has been done. In this sense, it is possible to speak a language without having studied its formal structure. The role of philosophy in the advancement of science is to make trouble: to challenge fundamental assumptions, to insist on rigor, and to demand some order of synoptic responsibility. It is not sufficient to *do*; it is also necessary to understand. In that spirit, we may say that psychiatry seeks philosophical comprehension whether or not individual psychiatrists follow that impulse. In dealing with the pathology of the person, the psychiatrist is, immanently at least, positing as well as probing the structure of the real. If phenomenology is not the ultimate instrument of psychiatric theory, it is at least a powerful reminder that without philosophy psychiatry cannot make a lasting claim to knowledge. Conversely, to the extent that its cardinal insight is valid, phenomenological philosophy is a precious clue to the nature of consciousness in its normal as well as pathological modalities.

E. W. S.
M. N.

Acknowledgment

I want to express my sincere thanks to the polyglot Lexingtonians: Dr. ERLING ENG, Clinical Psychologist at the Veterans Hospital, who translated my paper, and STEPHEN C. KENNEDY, student at the University of Kentucky Medical Center, who translated Professor EY's essay. My gratefulness and appreciation also belongs to Mrs. ANNE MANGOLD, Gilbertsville, New York, for her invaluable stylistic advice.

ERWIN W. STRAUS

Contents

HENRI EY :

Outline of an Organo-dynamic Conception of the Structure, Nosography, and Pathogenesis of Mental Diseases

Psychiatry and Philosophy

Erwin W. Straus

I. Introduction. Nature and Existence

Psychiatry is a branch of medicine. The professional training of the psychiatrist, like that of all other physicians, is controlled by the State, the practice of his profession State-supervised. Nevertheless, psychiatry cannot be easily fitted into the series of other specialties either limited to the treatment of particular organs or distinguished by the application of special procedures.

A hundred years ago, when GRIESINGER'S thesis, "mental illnesses are diseases of the brain", won general acceptance, the logical position of psychiatry within medicine and the natural sciences seemed unambiguously determined. Strangely enough, the term "psychiatry" began to gain currency at the very time when all psychic and intellectual accomplishments were interpreted as manifestations of localizable brain functions. That could happen only because "psyche" was identified in a naively casual manner with the brain, to such a degree that a hypothetical cerebral pathway of conduction was called the intrapsychic segment of the psychic reflex arc. The name "psychiatry" concealed the difficult task of separating the treatment of madness from that of neurological disorders, while at the same time bringing them together as psychiatry and neurology. "Enkephaliatry" would have been a more suitable term, if neurology had not established its priority. WERNICKE'S attempt to save the situation through a distinction of focal and diffuse brain disorders and to delineate "mental illnesses as expanded illnesses of the organ of association" was unsuccessful. With FREUD'S conceptualization of a psychic apparatus the precise boundaries of the organ area were of course widened or left indefinite; yet, at least in theory, FREUD remained true to the traditional principles. Psychotherapy, whether psychoanalytically oriented or not, whether practiced with or without a medical degree, emerged within psychiatry. While manual therapies determined surgery as a medical specialty—(surgery, i. e. chirurgy, literally means "hand-work")—psycho-therapy did not establish psychiatry.

Familiarity with neuro-anatomy, neuro-physiology, and neuro-pathology is still required today in the American Board examination in psychiatry. Nevertheless, during residency training, these "basic sciences" are often offered only in the third and last year of the curriculum—a tacit admission that they do not really function as basic sciences. Psychiatry is without a propaedeutic discipline of its own. In some continental hospitals psychiatry, neurology, and psychotherapy are still lodged together under one roof. But it is dubious whether this roof rests on one foundation. To silence our doubts we would need to know what essentially characterizes the mentally sick person, and, further, what distinguishes mental diseases from all the other diseases in such a basic manner that the specialty of psychiatry assumes a unique position in the field of medicine as a whole.

Since psychiatry is neither confined to the treatment of diseases of one organ nor restricted to one therapeutic technique, one may try to determine its peculiar character not by an attempt to establish boundaries but rather by the reverse, by recognizing the open horizon of its thematic field. While the activities of the physician are directed generally to man as a living creature, to the organism and its function, the psychiatrist is concerned with man as a citizen of the historical and social world or worlds. Psychiatric case histories are biographies in which parents are listed not only as progenitors, and brothers and sisters not only as siblings, but where they play their roles as members of a family to whom the patient has related and continues to relate himself in a particular way. The object of psychiatric action is not primarily the brain, the body, or the organism; it should be integral man in the uniqueness of his individual existence as this discloses itself—independently of the distinction between healthy and sick—in existential communication.

These inferences have been elaborated in the Dasein-analysis of LUDWIG BINSWANGER. "Psychiatry", BINSWANGER says, "is basically a science of man, of human existence"[1]. A psychiatrist, in his work, must be directed "to the encounter and mutal understanding with one's fellow man as a whole, and oriented to the understanding of man in his entirety..."[2].

Dasein-analysis however does not claim to represent the total structure of psychiatric knowledge. "It considers itself to be the handmaiden of clinical psychiatry... the real backbone of psychiatric medical science[3]." This ancillary role is, to be sure, not its primary task. In principle, Dasein-analysis is feasible without the psychiatric-clinical methods; it works at

---

[1] BINSWANGER, L.: Ausgewählte Vorträge und Aufsätze. S. 30. Bern: Francke-Verlag 1955.

[2] BINSWANGER, L.: Ausgewählte Vorträge und Aufsätze. S. 278. Bern: Francke-Verlag 1955.

[3] BINSWANGER, L.: Geleitwort zu HÄFNER, H.: Psychopathen. Berlin-Göttingen-Heidelberg: Springer 1961.

the *foundations* of the structure of psychiatry. The comparison between the life worlds of mentally sick and healthy persons sought for in existence-analysis is materially and methodically based on HEIDEGGER's phenomeno-logical-aprioric, ontological revealing of human existence and on HUSSERL's phenomenology of the transcendental constitution of consciousness.

BINSWANGER has been unwavering in his admiration for and gratitude to HEIDEGGER. Psychiatry in turn owes thanks to BINSWANGER for making accessible the endless riches of HEIDEGGER, who was successful "in reanimating the history of Western thought by an energetic and persistent return to 'the things themselves'" [1]. The intimate tie with the analytic of Dasein as worked out in "Being and Time" has however also turned out to be a burden for existence-analysis and through it for psychiatry.

HEIDEGGER, to be sure, did not, as FREUD did, come from or go into psychiatry. Even the opposition of authenticity and inauthenticity, i. e., "the possibility of existence to secure or to lose itself", is to be understood as an existential discrimination of modes of being, and not—as psycho-therapists most of all tend to believe—as a psychiatric description and evaluation. HEIDEGGER's rendering of "the they" (das Man) [2] leaves no doubt that the overwhelming majority of mankind, who neither suffer of themselves nor wrongfully cause others to suffer, live comfortably and contentedly in "the they".

"Proximally Dasein is 'they' and for the most part it remains so [3]." If inauthentic being were to be taken, not as *existentiale* but as a psychiatric category, then we psychiatrists would have to invite all mankind into our offices, with the presumptuous attitude that, by reason of our training, we had become successful not only in realizing our own selves but in helping others to do the same. "But the inauthenticity of Dasein does not signify any 'less' Being or any 'lower' degree of Being. Rather it is the case that even in its fullest concretion Dasein can be characterized by inauthenticity—when busy, when excited, when interested, when ready for enjoyment [4]." Therefore, a brief critical evaluation is required not only to justify our own formulations but also to save what has been won by Dasein-analysis for psychiatry, present and to come.

HEIDEGGER's analytic of Dasein, which takes the ordinary everyday world—"proximally and for the most part"—as its point of departure,

---

[1] KARL LÖWITH: Heidegger, Denker in dürftiger Zeit. Frankfurt a. M.: S. Fischer 1953.

[2] It has been suggested (RICHARDSON) that HEIDEGGER's "das Man" is best rendered by "people". But for the sake of the reader who may be familiar with HEIDEGGER only from English translation, the terminology of the standard translation of "Being and Time" by JOHN MACQUARRIE and EDWARD ROBINSON (Harper & Row, 1962) is here followed throughout. — E. E.

[3] Being and Time, p. 167.

[4] Being and Time, p. 68.

serves a higher task; it is devoted to finding an answer to the question of the "meaning of Being". *Human* everydayness is chosen as theme because man, amid all that is, is distinguished by the fact "that, in its very Being, that Being is an *issue* for it ... that Dasein, in its Being, has a relationship towards that Being ... that with and through its Being this Being is disclosed to it"[1]. That which is (das Seiende) in the human mode of Being is termed Dasein, "that kind of Being towards which Dasein can comport itself in one way or the other, and always comports itself somehow, we call 'existence'"[2].

Thus HEIDEGGER most emphatically separates that which is—the ontic—from Being which is not ontic. "Dasein is ontically distinctive in that it *is* ontological[3]." Because of this interlacing of ontic and ontological, "the human mode of being" is destined to become the object of an ontological investigation. For in every explication of that which is, "Being, that which determines the ontic as ontic" is already somehow understood.

HEIDEGGER's own anticipatory understanding of Being, which, guiding the analytic from the very start, is to be explicated through the analytic, brings him into opposition to the entire tradition of Western philosophy, which HEIDEGGER reproaches with "forgetfulness of Being". Ignoring the "ontological difference", philosophical thought, soon after its beginning in Greek antiquity, turned away from meditation on the meaning of Being and toward an exploration of that which is. "In the ontology of the ancients, the entities we encounter within the world are taken as the basic examples for the interpretation of Being[4]."

In turning thus to physical things, traditional philosophy made the "present-at-hand" with its corresponding temporal order become the sole prevailing mode of Being. In "Being and Time" existence—the mode of Being of Dasein—is presented in sharp contrast to the mode of Being of the "present-at-hand". Corresponding to this separation of Dasein from everything else that lacks the character of Dasein is HEIDEGGER's opposition of his own freshly minted concept of existentialia (Existenzialien) to the traditional concept of categories, or rather the subordination of these to those. The definition of the Being of Dasein takes place through the existentialia; the definition of that which is, but which has not the character of Dasein, takes place through the categories. Presence-at-hand and existence are "the two basic possibilities for characters of Being ... any entity is either a 'who' (existence) or a 'what' (presence-at-hand in the broadest sense)"[5].

---

[1] Being and Time, p. 32.
[2] Being and Time, p. 32.
[3] Being and Time, p. 32.
[4] Being and Time, p. 70.
[5] Being and Time, p. 71.

Since, according to HEIDEGGER, in traditional anthropology the Being of Man has been "taken for granted" in the sense of being present-at-hand like the other things of creation, the distinction of modes of Being allows the question "what is man?" to be raised anew and to be newly answered in the analytic of Dasein. BINSWANGER's Dasein-analysis has made its findings available to psychiatry, a contribution that remains unaffected even if BINSWANGER's adoption of Heideggerian ideas was based on a "productive misunderstanding" [1] rather than on a legitimate extrapolation. Yet we may wonder whether an acceptance of the first issue obligates us in this case to subscribe to the entire work. I do not believe that it does, nor do I believe that any regional ontology fruitful for medicine and psychiatry can be developed from the fundamental ontology of HEIDEGGER. The analytic of Dasein remains a massive torso; it lacks any tie with life, nature, and lived body (Leib), in short with the "animalia" that are indispensable for founding an anthropology and a human nosology. This fact cannot have remained hidden from HEIDEGGER himself, for he has in his later works repeatedly rejected an anthropological interpretation of "Being and Time". His own position therefore supports a criticism of "Being and Time" as a presumptively anthropological or even psychopathological-anthropological work.

The analytic of Dasein is dominated by the idea of existence. Just as FREUD, at the close of "The Interpretation of Dreams", apostrophized consciousness by asking: "What role remains in our presentation for the once almighty consciousness?" and answered, "Only that of a sense organ for the perception of psychic qualities", so HEIDEGGER might have asked: "What role remains in our presentation for the once almighty all-else-concealing presence-at-hand?" In the enthusiasm of discovery all light is focussed on the *existentialia* and what is present-at-hand is placed in the shadow. Consequently only that much of Dasein is taken into consideration as can be accommodated to the program of hermeneutic interpretation; or phenomena that are not uniquely human are nevertheless existentially interpreted in the sense of an anticipatory understanding of Being. To give an example: a brief characterization of "Being-in" opens the chapter on "Being-in-the-world" as the basic constitution of Dasein. "Being-in" is conceived as the formal, existential expression of the Being of Dasein. Is this delimitation to man justifiable? Doesn't "Being-in" also apply to te bird "who dwells the leafy twigs among" or to the fox who leaves his lair by one exit and returns by another? And doesn't "Being-alongside" apply to the dog who follows his master? Does man's "Being-in" originate in the Being of Dasein, or does it originate, for man and animal alike, in their animal nature?

[1] Compare BINSWANGER's remark concerning his Heidegger interpretation in his book *Grundformen und Erkenntnis des menschlichen Daseins.* Zürich: Max Niehans Verlag 1942: Preface to the fourth edition. München. 1964.

The dichotomy of the modes of Dasein, in its claim to be complete, opens up a hiatus. The universe of all that is, is divided into two unequal realms. On this side of the dividing line stands man interpreted as Dasein. Everything else that is, atoms and galaxies as well as stones, plants, and animals, are placed on the other side of the gulf. Thereby, however, a void is created into which the terrain that is proper to medicine and psychiatry threatens to disappear. The "ready-to-hand" may well be included in the sphere of "presence-at-hand" in its broadest sense. But how is the Being of animals to be understood? And how is man as *zoon*, as animal, to be comprehended? Ontically viewed, man is a living being who shares conception and death, breathing and eating, waking and sleeping, movement and sensory orientation, with the animal. The difference between man and animal cannot obliterate their kinship. Comprehension of the living body cannot be derived from existence (Existenz). The radical separation of modes of being prevents an account of man in his corporeality and as a person; it obscures his relationship to the animals and to nature; in short, it prevents the understanding of man as creature. Yet health and sickness certainly are manifestations of men and animals as living creatures.

With the distinction of the modes of Being the question arises of the possibility of their reunification, not limited to the modes of Being themselves but in relation also to the ontic regions determined by them. Man can put his hand on that which is present-at-hand; he sets his foot on the supporting ground; through inhaling and exhaling he remains in uninterrupted exchange with the surrounding nature. Modes of Being may be distinguished more easily than united conceptually, since after all their unification is possible only in a "higher" mode of Being, present in everything that is. But the problem is not limited to comprehending how "Dasein" and the present-at-hand are able to enter into communication. The ontic and the modes of Being are not neatly separated; man is a being determined not simply by *one* kind of Being. He has a body (Körper); he is lived body (Leib), animal, creature, and existence. There is no point in denying that the merely present-at-hand is only secondarily discovered in the everyday world; yet it is discovered as something "already there", not as something that is first constituted through the discovery. Even if it should be the case that the theoretical attitude of cognition—at times scorned by Heidegger as a "frozen staring at the present-at-hand"—were a deficient mode compared with the attitude of circumspect caring, does this imply that presence-at-hand is a deficient kind of Being, comparable, say, to matter in the Plotinian doctrine of emanation?

In "Being and Time" there are only a few references to the ontological problem of "life", and these confuse rather than clarify. "Life, in its own right, is a kind of Being; but essentially it is accessible only in Dasein. The ontology of life is accomplished by way of a privative interpretation; it determines what must be the case if there can be anything like mere-aliveness. Life is not a mere Being-present-at-hand, nor is it Dasein" [1]. How this "neither-nor" can be converted into "as-well-as" is not explained, nor can it be explained. HEIDEGGER categorically rejects a theory of levels. "Dasein is never to be defined ontologically by regarding it as life (in an ontologically indefinite manner) plus something else." The situation somehow reminds us of DESCARTES' fruitless efforts to comprehend man as a composite of two different substances. That life is essentially accessible in Dasein does not distinguish it from all other themes to which thinking man is able to turn; that life, or better still, the realm of living creatures, can be reached only through a private interpretation will find assent neither in science nor in everyday life.

The paucity of comments concerning life is remarkable in a book containing such profound meditations about death. The discussions of death are, to be sure, devoted to its existential interpretation, which, HEIDEGGER asserts, takes precedence over all biology and ontology of life [2]. But even the existential interpretation must recognize death as a "phenomenon of life." Dasein can assume an attitude toward its death only because man, like all animals, is born, lives, and dies. In this chapter HEIDEGGER just repeats, with only a few additions, his earlier explications. "Life", he now says, "must be understood as a kind of Being to which there belongs a Being-in-the-world. Only if this kind of Being is oriented in a privative way to Dasein can we fix its character ontologically. Even Dasein may be considered purely as life" [3]. But how can Being-in-the-world belong to life, since Being-in-the-world after all characterizes the constitution of the Being of Dasein? HEIDEGGER has not shown how the privative orientation is to be enacted. It appears to be a mode of observation that certainly does not constitute life, but, at best, reveals what life is. There are good reasons to wonder how a privative orientation could bring to light what is initially hidden. The privation must certainly somehow extend to the Being-in-the-world itself, so that "pure life" appears as a residual, as a sort of intermediate realm between presence-at-hand and existence. Thus considered as "pure life", Dasein "passes" into that domain of Being that we know as the world of plants and animals, "a field in which we can obtain data about life's duration, propagation, and growth" [4]. The summary coercion of the world of plants and animals into a single domain of Being, to which, purely as life, Dasein is also said to belong, not only ignores the differences between plants and animals but also the features common to animals and man. This attitude is amazing, all the more so because all existential doing

---

[1] Being and Time, p. 75.
[2] Being and Time, p. 291.
[3] Being and Time, p. 290.
[4] Being and Time, p. 290.

and suffering occur on a basis common to steed and rider, that of primary
sensory orientation and of movement.

Together with the domain of the purely vital, the realm of medical
research and practice also appears to be delineated. Obviously, HEIDEGGER
is not entirely satisfied with this result, for he raises the question: "Or
must sickness and death in general—even from a medical point of view—
be primarily conceived as existential phenomena?" [1] The wording and the
prominence of the question at the end of a paragraph that deals with ending, perishing, and dying, suggest a positive answer to the reader. It seems
to me that BINSWANGER in his analyses of Dasein has assumed this position.
All the cases classified as schizophrenic in the psychiatric clinic must be
understood as disturbances in the progress and realization of Dasein. The
interpretation of Dasein-analysis is said to be "indifferent to the concepts
of healthy and sick, of normal and abnormal" [2].

The nosological categories of the clinic are replaced by development and
structures of Dasein, held together by their inner consistency. These cases
are, to be sure, interpreted Dasein-analytically not just as medical cases but
as failures of existential projects. Therefore, the findings of Dasein-analysis
must be translated into the language of the clinic as a second step. However,
such a pluralistic interpretation remains unsatisfactory [3]. It stems from a
tendency to consider existence as absolute over against life, a separation
unacceptable to psychiatry.

HEIDEGGER, as already mentioned, has left open the question of an
existential interpretation of sickness, although the original distinction
between modes of Being suggests an affirmative response. Nevertheless,
unqualified affirmation that is not limited to neuroses runs counter to the
fact that Dasein ends when life comes to a close through illness, violent
injury, or exhaustion from age, since all this happens likewise to animals—
at times even from diseases contagious for humans. Dasein can accept death
as its extreme possibility, but only as a possibility inherent in life itself.

The analytic of Dasein interprets everydayness as "that Being which is
'between' birth and death" [4]. Medicine considers a broader scope, namely
that between *conception* and death—not out of pedantry or a picayune
concern with facts; if for no other reason, clinical experience with hereditary
illnesses and malformations makes it mandatory. Here the psychiatrist must
face natural conditions that keep the individual from realizing his basic
possibilities or, under favorable conditions, enable him to realize them.
Birth and death are the beginning and the end of the individual life of man,

[1] Being and Time, p. 291.
[2] BINSWANGER, L.: Schizophrenie. Pfullingen: Neske 1957.
[3] Cf. HÄFNER, H.: Psychopathen. Berlin-Göttingen-Heidelberg: Springer 1961.
[4] Being and Time, p. 276.

who matures from child to adult through a process of growth that is no achievement of his own. Birth and death are related to each other as the beginning and the end of the individual life. Such an analogy does not exist between procreation and death. In procreation, the individual life arises from parts in the continuity of generations; in death it breaks down, it ends with Being-no-more. Its starting and ending are not finite in the same way. Death and dying may be elucidated by the dialectic of Being and Nothingness. Procreation and birth cannot be conceived in the same antithesis. Fertilization itself is inaccessible to human action. One can interfere with it, prevent it, but no one can make it. We have all been engendered as natural sons and daughters. As we move back, then, from birth to procreation this ontologically significant question forces itself upon us: Since "the entity . . . which we are ourselves" [1] is generated by its parents, is Being co-generated? The natural start is more puzzling than the natural finish. As generated and as generating, the "simple organism" is more, not less than Dasein. Man knows about his generation; as a rule he knows those who have generated him and who recognize him as their offshoot, so that he can enter as an heir into the historical succession of generations. The natural sequence of the generations establishes the basis of the historical order of ancestors and descendants. From the natural family arises the human family, to which the individual in his existence belongs as a member.

The generation and emergence of man—of every human being—is subject to biological law. The generation of just *this* particular human being is, in a certain sense, accidental. A man and a woman, a sperm and an ovum, had to join; not this man and that woman, nor this cell and that cell. Astrology was, of course, one attempt to subordinate the contingent character of generation to the lawfulness of cosmic patterns. As a *living* human being each one is an instance of the genus. As a living *human* being, each one enters the space of historical Dasein independently equipped for this journey with his own possibilities and their limitations. Measured by the standard of HEIDEGGER's style, and compared with his, as it were, clairvoyant certitude, the sparse references to "life" are surprising in their ambiguity, their indecisiveness and contradictions, indicating that the problem has not been resolved. If being sick cannot be understood existentially, then the problems are reversed. The ontic qualification of man as *zoon* obliges us to reflect about what it is that makes it possible for this creature to be privileged with historical existence and what the circumstances are that alienate him from his destiny. In his later works HEIDEGGER named man "the herdsman of Being". Does he first become human after receiving this call, or does Being call and e-voke him because his nature has fitted him to meet such a challenge?

---

[1] Being and Time, p. 67.

The neutrality of Dasein-analysis with regard to the distinctions of normal and abnormal, healthy and sick, is not an arbitrary attitude; it is imposed by the notion of mineness (Jemeinigkeit), which actually frustrates all attempts to establish a norm. We must wonder whether even the attempt to describe the course of a single Dasein must not fail, insofar as the statement "individuum est ineffabile" is taken as valid. According to Heidegger, mineness, just like existence, is a characteristic of Being and not of the entities. "The Being of any such entity (which we ourselves are) is in each case mine [1]." Thus may the two pillar statements that open the presentation of the Analytic of Dasein be united. The Being of Dasein in its transcendence is the possibility of the most radical individuation. There repeatedly occur formulations like: "These entities, in their Being, comport themselves toward their Being", an expression which appears to point to a pluralism of Being [2]. Nevertheless, since Dasein *is* its own possibility, it can never be ontologically interpreted as "an instance or special case of some genus of entities as things that are present-at-hand" [3]. Consequently Dasein does not denote the human being as we are used to speaking of man—or more precisely of men—in everyday life and in medicine. In spite of such emphasis on radical individuation, the theme of the analytic of Dasein is the structure of the Being of this entity in its full generic sense. Differences in human life histories play no part; Dasein is not synonymous with man. The analytic of Dasein ascends, to be sure, towards a position where the question of the meaning of Being can be answered; but man as Dasein has already been interpreted in looking backwards from that goal. Thus the title of "Dasein" does not express its "what", but rather its Being. The theme of the analytic is not human creatures but the being whose essence lies in its "to be". In a later work Heidegger says, "In order to denote the linkage of Being to the essence of man, as well as the essential relation of man to the openness ("there") of Being as such, together in one word, the name "Dasein" was selected for the domain of essence in which man stands as man" [4]. Dasein, then, does not designate the human being but is the name of the domain of essence. Since in Heidegger ascent to Being is always already pre-interpreted as a descent from Being, he sees no material contradiction between the later interpretation of the essence of man as the "there of Being" and the original terminology in the analytic of Dasein. Although the analytic of the Dasein of man starts from his everydayness, still it moves ever farther and farther away from the "life world" of human beings.

---

[1] Being and Time, p. 67.
[2] Being and Time, p. 67.
[3] Being and Time, p. 67—68.
[4] Heidegger, M.: Was ist Metaphysik: 5. Aufl. Frankfurt a. M.: Klostermann 1949. Transl. by E. E.

The expression "Dasein" conceals many implicit difficulties. The German word "Dasein" is neuter, sexless, without plural; it is an abstract, impersonal, objectivating term. Dasein is an *it* in common usage, not a *he* or a *she,* and definitely not a "thou" or an "I".

It remains to be considered whether this neutrality is non-essential and does not influence the analytic itself. Formulations that fit *the* Dasein, *the* (das) ontic, *the* (das) Being, can scarcely be applied to the (der) man, the (die) woman, *the* (das) child. The individual human is typically non-whole, not only with regard to temporality and history but already through the biologically fundamental difference between the sexes and generations. No one man is the man. The new-born baby is a boy or a girl. Each is moietic in the sense of the Aristophanic myth. From the union of man and woman, of male and female cells, springs, nevertheless, a being, not-whole in the natural sense. This natural, sexually bound, "not-whole being" opens to man possibilities of entering into relations of sexual symbiosis and thereby of generations where authentic being no longer occurs in solitary confrontation with nothingness. Dasein, in the analytic, is neither male nor female, neither young nor old. Dasein is a term for the entity of the mode of Being: man. Psychiatry however, is not concerned with *man* but with men in their natural, conditioned character. The creature who has emerged from the act of generation lives on, growing older continually, and that also means he is determined by his past. He doesn't create himself. His existence, his historicality, are supported and made possible by his living body but are also threatened from there.

The boundaries of possible realization that precede all self-realization are not established by the self. The boundaries drawn for man as a living being also establish the alternatives of being sick or being well. Health, demanding optimal regulations, is thus endangered in many ways. The one health must prevail over the many modes of being sick. To be exposed to disease is a human inheritance. Sicknesses are natural, typical possibilities of the individual. The individual falls sick insofar as he is a member of the human species. The individual becomes sick "by nature". Whether mental illness or particular psychoses do not conform to the natural order is a question that must still be considered.

Anticipating the charge of having omitted "nature" from "Being and Time", HEIDEGGER wrote, "nature is to be met with neither in the circle of the surroundings nor at all as primarily something to which we relate ourselves" [1]. To describe the surroundings "in which Dasein maintains itself proximally and for the most part" [2] HEIDEGGER used the world of the craftsman as a model. But does the characterization of "proximally" really

---

[1] HEIDEGGER, M.: Vom Wesen des Grundes. 3. Aufl. Frankfurt a. M.: Klostermann 1949. Transl. by E. E.

[2] Being and Time, p. 153.

fit? Dasein does not enter a workshop already fully equipped; it has been
built by human beings, created in their struggle with nature. Always present
are the "elements which hate what human hands have formed" (SCHILLER),
the elements which man had first to yoke. Within nature man turns against
nature, using the gifts and strengths she has given him. The man-made
surroundings do not arise from mere adaptation to nature, nor from using
what is ready-to-hand, but from being produced. Prometheus brought man
the fire he had stolen from heaven. But men could not have used it if they
had not understood how to control the flame. Material, too, must be
provided; the living tree is converted into wood (hyle) only by the blows
of the axe. The tree is con-verted into human use, i. e., di-verted from the
natural order into an alien one but one fitting human purpose. To chop
down trees and cut then up, men need the tools they have invented. It is
these that mediate between the nature of things and the nature of man.
All of them are composed so that one part is fitted to the human body—the
handle, for "handling", the other part to the "thing at hand". As in contemporary houses electric switches are made so that the combination of
conducting and nonconducting parts permits us to manipulate the electric
circuit with impunity, so pokers make it possible to stir the fire and hammer
and tongs to forge the glowing iron.

But HEIDEGGER does not need to hear these things from someone else.
The situation of the "naked savage" is not omitted incidentally; it is intentionally skipped. HEIDEGGER enumerates a number of reasons why he did
not take the world of the primitives but rather the shop of the manual
worker as the or a model for his analysis of the surrounding. But his explanation is not enough to silence doubts whether the order of "proximally"
and "subsequently" in his impressive treatment of the surrounding has not
been reversed and whether the artificial surroundings have not been given
priority over natural surroundings. "In roads, streets, bridges, buildings",
HEIDEGGER says, "our concern discovers Nature as having some definite
direction [1]." An explorer, however, who comes upon remnants of walks,
bridges, and buildings, in a remote and trackless waste, concludes that man
must once have lived in that inaccessible region. Human artifacts arise on
the ground of "untouched" nature. In its deliberate effort to challenge and
reverse this obvious order, analysis of the surroundings aims at revealing
"circumspect provision", "referential networks" and "readiness-to-hand"
of "equipment". This opens the way for the interpretation of the historicality of Dasein. Linked with this tendency to present existence as the essence
of Dasein is the opposite tendency to represent presence-at-hand as a
derivative mode. HEIDEGGER intends to show that what is present-at-hand
is met with originally in the human surroundings. "Readiness-to-hand is the

---

[1] Being and Time, p. 100.

way in which entities as they are 'in themselves' are defined ontologico-categorically [1]." "To lay bare what is just present-at-hand and no more, cognition must first penetrate *beyond* what is ready-to-hand in our concern [2]." Only in looking aside from the readiness-to-hand, Heidegger claims, does one discover nature in its pure presence-at-hand. If the present-at-hand were actually discovered from the ready-to-hand as a deficient mode, then the artificial surroundings of the workshop would necessarily have to be put "proximally" before the natural surroundings.

The dubiousness of identifying nature with the present-at-hand becomes especially clear in the discussion of materials from which an artifact is produced. A product, for example, a shoe, is said to refer back to leather, leather to hides, and hides to the animals from which they have been taken. Animals are raised, "but also occur within the world without having been raised at all ... So in the environment certain entities become accessible which are always ready-to-hand, but which, in themselves, do not need to be produced ... In equipment that is used, 'Nature' is by that use discovered—the 'Nature' we find in natural products" [3]. But this happens only in the land of Cockaigne: Animals do not of their own will bring their skins to market; they must be tamed, raised, and finally killed. Or they must be obtained by the hunter or trapper through dangerous struggle, using insight which corresponds to the theoretical attitude in which things are observed at a distance and in their particular character. The final product, the shoes, indeed refer back to the materials, that is to say, when considered by a reflective spectator. In the process of manufacturing, however, the referential networks must first be established, often even by force.

The grazing cattle and the wild game, which must first be killed, do not refer to shoes, any more than the tusks of an attacking elephant refer to chess figures, the fleece of unborn lambs to fur coats, or pitchblende to atomic bombs. Through the anticipating gaze of man animals must be forced into a referential linkage determined by possible usage. For the hunter lying in wait the prey is in no sense of the word "ready-to-hand", any more than is the wood for the settler clearing the primeval forest with fire and axe. In short, the material does not refer to its use, but must be initially acquired by man in order to be used. Primitive techniques are like those more advanced ones in that they violently interfere with a natural context in order to provide material for one quite different. In this process all action is guided by a preceding insight. In order to trick the wild animal with his snares and to bring it into his power, alive or dead, the hunter must in a preparatory phase refrain from all active intervention. Covertly he must first discover the rules of the animal's behavior, in order to arrange his ruses

---

[1] Being and Time, p. 101.
[2] Being and Time, p. 101.
[3] Being and Time, p. 100.

accordingly. From the fact "that knowing is grounded beforehand in a Being-already-alongside-the-world" [1] it does not follow that knowing is a deficient mode, nor that it is a staring at a pure eidos. Such a staring at the purely present-at-hand would certainly be of little use for action. "Uncircumspect just looking-at" would never lead from the domestication of cattle to the obtaining of leather. The farmer who drives his animals out to pasture *knows* very well why he does so. Anticipatorily reflecting, he knows that he will be able to remove their hides later. He inserts the animals he meets in the pasture into an altogether different con-text: the production and sale of leather. He compels the beasts to enter into a nexus to which they do not refer of themselves. Nonetheless he does not view the cattle as merely present-at-hand, even if he deals with them as beasts, which is to say that he does not respect them in their own being as living creatures. Perhaps the Greeks called "things" *pragmata* not because they dealt with them in a "concerned" way, but because, in contradistinction to the natural formations of *physis,* they were initially produced by human *praxis.*

Human beings erect the workshop as their surround in a struggle with nature. HEIDEGGER is unwilling to admit that nature may be encountered as Might. "The wood is a forest of timber, the mountain a quarry of rock; the river is water-power, the wind is wind 'in the sails' [2]." Yet the river becomes water-power only when the water has been successfully led to the mill, and sails swell in the wind only after the *invention,* not the finding, of boats and sails. But winds are fickle; man can make use of them only when they are favorable; the sailor is continually exposed to calms, gales and counter-currents. As he is dependent on the winds, so the farmer is on the rain and sun, over which he has no power. The merely present-at-hand—for example, water measured and sold by the cubic foot—is not, however, the nature in which man originally found himself, the nature which supports and threatens him, a power embodied in the animal divinities. In GOETHE's verse: "Earth, thou too, This night persisteth through . . ." [3], the earth is not addressed as present-at-hand or as ready-to-hand, but as the well-founded, enduring Earth, as the ground which refers to nothing else, and from which every question of "what for" glances off. Only the ontological difference transforms the ontic—addressed grammatically in the form of the participle as Seiend (or)—into something characterized through the mode of Being of presence-at-hand. The purely present-at-hand is a construction of mathematical science; it is not, however, the sole possible alternative to the ready-to-hand and to Dasein.

The man-made surroundings of the workshop have been wrested from nature by a constant struggle. These surroundings are not those of Dasein

---

[1] Being and Time, p. 88.
[2] Being and Time, p. 100.
[3] Goethe: Faust, pt. II. Transl. by E. E.

but of men; they are populated by masters, journeymen, and apprentices. The younger generation must first learn from the older how to handle the tools. The statement:"We come across equipment for writing, sewing, working, transportation, measurement" [1], holds true only for the grandchild whose forefathers invented such equipment, who did not find it already present. In "Being and Time" the ontological interpretation of the world takes precedence; only subsequently is the question of "Who" raised, a question supposed to point to the "they" *(Man)* as resident of the world of everyday. Yet just as Dasein does not denote a human, but rather his essence (as existence), so the "they" does not characterize the men who, in the confines of the workshop, are complementarily related to one another as masters and servants, as owners and employees, or as teachers and students.

Manual skills must be acquired by the young because the human surroundings are man-made, they are artificial. The handling of equipment *must* be learned, and that presupposes that it can be learned. The master of a craft must combine know-how and manual skill. The apprentice learns to make the tools serve him, while he, in a certain way, serves them until he finally masters them and embodies them into his own body activity. He learns to saw and to plane, as he moves *himself* in the way that the saw and plane demand to be moved. Everything that man performs in his surroundings is, in the last analysis, rooted in the fact that he is able, as body subject, to move with sight and hearing in the world, and thus to relate himself to the surroundings, to other human beings, and to himself.

The question of whether a suitable interpretation has been assigned to the body subject and body subjectness in the analytic of Dasein remains a moot one. BINSWANGER and others claim that within the explication of the *existentiale* of thrownness "Dasein as bodily presence is always co-implied" [2]. Nevertheless the very expression "thrownness" shows that the body subject is experienced as a burden, a boundary, a fate, just like the "Da" (there), into which Dasein finds itself flung. In this interpretation the body is not the lived, supporting body, not the body of a man who walks, stands, jumps, and acts. Nor is that body the lived body of the man who sees. In the section on "Being-here as State-of-mind" another reference is made to seeing as a staring-at. There HEIDEGGER says, "Indeed from the *ontological point of view* we must as a general principle leave the primary discovery of the world to 'bare mood'. Pure beholding, even if it were to penetrate to the innermost core of the Being of something present-at hand, could never discover anything like that which is threatening" [3]. But seeing in the primary orientation is not pure beholding, just as a man in living

---

[1] Being and Time, p. 97.
[2] BINSWANGER, L.: Vorträge und Aufsätze, II, S. 270 (Transl. by E. E.).
[3] Being and Time, p. 177.

movement does not experience himself only as "state-of-mind determined". With the term "thrownness" the body subject is interpreted as if it were an incarnation forced upon Dasein. "Has Dasein as itself ever decided freely whether it wants to come into 'Dasein' or not, and will it ever be able to make such a decision? [1]" Yet only a "finished" being, flung from nothingness into "there" (Da), can so decide and so question; a man of flesh and blood cannot, neither an adult who worries about his ancestry, nor a child who, growing up with and in his lived body, experiences the unfolding of his life space. The human infant, born physiologically prematurely, must, according to PORTMANN, first learn how to carry out his natural functions like walking, standing, and talking. He doesn't learn walking from the grown-ups, even if he does so with their help. In speaking, however, he must adopt language from others. In learning, the child enters into the order of the social surroundings in which he historically "exists".

In the attitude of daily life, as in scientific reflection, man is first of all a creature of blood and flesh who casts a shadow and yet can leap over his own shadow. Psychiatry, which deals with disturbances of human behavior, asks whether and how far the disturbances it observes, describes, and treats, are conditioned by sicknesses, i. e., by failures of natural performance in the broadest sense of the word. One of its fundamental problems is the relation of nature and historical existence, already pointed out in BINSWANGER's distinction of vital functions and inner life history. In the past it had been difficult for psychiatry, with its attachment to science, to make sense out of the leap over the shadow. The analytic of Dasein was an act of liberation. Nevertheless, returning now from the ontological interpretation, we still have the task of assigning to being-in-the-world a position that is gravity-bound and within the whole of nature. Psychiatry, which deals with sickness, requires a solution for the problem from philosophy. Actually the question of the norm takes priority over questions of the possibilities of disturbances, even though it is clinical experience that first of all forces us to ask such questions.

"Being and Time" was published in 1927. At that time the young interns now in our clinics had not been born, and men who are today in their fifties were still in school. HEIDEGGER produced his masterpiece in the middle of his life. Ever since then he has meditated untiringly on the question of the "meaning of Being", taking up over and over again the relation of man to Being. His changes of view need not occupy us here, since BINSWANGER's Dasein-analysis has remained true to HEIDEGGER's analytic of Dasein in "Being and Time". Questions of method, like those concerning the relation of HEIDEGGER's hermeneutic phenomenology to the transcendental phenomenology of HUSSERL, may also be passed over. Above all HEIDEGGER's

---

[1] Being and Time, p. 271.

ontology has concerned us here insofar as, through Dasein-analysis, it has influenced psychiatry itself. And yet one more question at issue should be briefly considered in concluding this opening section.

Dasein-analysis demands that the psychiatrist encounter the patient as a fellow human being, wholly, in a genuinely communicative relation. Psychiatric practice is far from meeting this requirement; but there are good reasons for its failure.

Medical communication with a patient cannot be without reservation for the simple reason that one physician deals with many patients to whom he allots but a portion of his professional time and that for monetary compensation. How could he ever understand the other wholly except by giving himself up to him?

No one expects of a psychiatrist that, in existential communication, he should adopt the patient's delusional ideas. Even in the momentous encounter of two individuals, each partner sinks back again and again into the shadow of the "he" or "she". The distance of objectivation is not an existential betrayal of the sick person; it is the indispensable condition of psychiatric activity. That an "I-he" relation cannot be transformed into one of "I and thou" is a primary, lifeworld manifestation of psychosis. To uncover its basis remains our task.

Medicine deals with "cases". The healing art made the knowledge of healing serve it. But medical knowledge can be taught and learned only if it formulates its knowledge as propositions which, obligatory for all, are valid in many single cases. BINSWANGER's Dasein-analyses have been deliberately presented as "The Case of Ellen West", "The Case of Jürg Zünd". These names obviously designate the patient as he or she is to be addressed in society in the third person. Of course that does not say whether they are to be understood as cases of a particular nosological category or of a particular disturbance of the order of Dasein.

In his practice the psychiatrist does not meet the patient as a fellow man whom he subsequently reduces to a clinical case. Occasionally the reverse may occur. The psychiatrist encounters a sick person and, to be sure, a sick person of particular sort. In the paradigmatic instance of a severe psychosis, the sick person must put up with the fact of being forced to see a doctor and to submit to treatment. As we say, the mental patient lacks insight into his condition. Health and *eudaemonia* have different meanings in psychiatry than they have elsewhere in medicine, where *eudaemonia*, "the good life", appears in contrast to the experience of suffering, pain, and bodily failure. Ailing and dis-ease—not diseases—form the prime experience that asks the healing arts for cure, i. e., for care and attention. Sickness has been discovered by the suffering patients, not by the physician. The sick person feels badly, feels ill (i. e. evil); he notices that "something is wrong". Asking for help, to be made well again, he turns to the physician, who has learned to order dis-ease into diseases and to recognize their manifestations, origins, and courses, and knows how to treat them. The mentally sick person suffers too, but he does not interpret his suffering as a failure conditioned by the body. He suffers from the malice of the world. In colloquial language the psychiatrist's patient is not recognized as "sick", but as "off his rocker", as "out of his head", or as "not quite right". The hospital psychiatrist who accepts such a person, who keeps him on a locked ward and declares him "incompetent", crosses, in his judgment and decisions, the boundaries otherwise respected in everyday-life medicine. The psychiatrist treats his patients, frequently acting for them and often enough against them; he will do everything in his power to prevent a suicidal patient from carrying out his intention. The medical relationship to the mentally sick person requires precisely that the patient be evaluated as such and be cared for with the caution and concern his sickness requires, without making him responsible for his acts. In his clinical work the psychiatrist implicitly assumes an attitude toward the philosophical problems of self-determination and of normal and morbid behavior. From such decisions he cannot withdraw; philosophical problems thrust themselves upon him. The position he takes may in the individual case be limited to action that follows accepted doctrines and rules of the art; or he may attempt to make philosophical questions thematic and to answer them in his clinical attitude. EUGEN BLEULER's "Natural History of the Soul" is an example. A third possibility is to become a student of the philosophers and to base psychiatry on philosophical work, as JASPERS did, even before BINSWANGER. With his distinctions between process and development, causal and intelligible connections, static and genetic understanding, as well as in his emphasis on method, JASPERS tried to render the philosophical ideas of DILTHEY, WINDELBAND, and RICKERT useful for psychiatry. But methodic rigor and the transfer of ideas from the history of philosophy to psychiatry have also had an inhibiting effect. With the reference to intuitive "presentification" of individual experience and empathy (Vergegenwärtigung of JASPERS), one of the basic problems, if not the basic problem, of psychiatry, the issue of the possibility of communication and comprehension, is bypassed.

II. Communication and the Common

Instead of proceeding from philosophy to psychiatry we shall start from psychiatry and let it lead us to philosophical questions. Thus I shall apply a kind of philosophical *"epoche"*, i. e., I will first bracket all philosophical teachings (as far as they are known to me) and launching out from the psychiatric situation I shall expose myself to philosophical adventures, with the risk of incurring the scorn of experts. I shall scan clinical experience for its hidden content of philosophical problems and attempt to propose a solution for some of the problems uncovered in the perusal.

As a psychiatrist, a certain position and role has been prescribed for me in the everyday human world. I conduct myself as one of many whose specialty has assigned to them certain tasks and modes of behavior. I can of course meditate at any time on myself, my role in society, and my relation to the world and to nature, but only insofar as I interrupt my actual psychiatric activity. In psychiatric practice I accept the order of the everyday human world and cooperate actively in its realization. I address myself to a particular group of fellow men, namely those in need of help, insofar as they have failed in undisturbed co-enactment of everyday life's meaningful requirements. Psychiatry is concerned with the means and ways of providing help; helplessness itself it did not discover. Psychiatry is a young discipline, but acquaintance with madness is ancient. Even if we did not have evidence like the Biblical stories of the possession of King Saul or the Sophoclean tragedy of mad Ajax, we would still be certain that the experience of madness is as old as mankind itself. Delusion is not restricted to particular times and places. Whether madness is seen as a curse or as a blessing, as possession or as inspiration, as guilt or as illness, all such views are based on an encounter with human beings with whom all mutual understanding flounders, because their own standpoint in the world is deranged.

"Strangeness" is the practical criterion for our distinction of mental disease from mental health. The psychiatrist ("alienist") (and not only he) interprets the "strange" behavior ("alienation") as a manifestation of sickness. In what particular sense the sick persons are "strange" need not be conceptually clear. Just as we discover a foreigner in the course of a conversation by his accent, i. e. by its contrast to that familiar to us, and just as we notice grammatical errors without being familiar with the rules of grammar, except in applying them, so the strangeness is realized as a fact, even though it is not understood in its structure. What we directly experience in the "life world" is the failure of mutual understanding; only through reflection do we arrive at conceptual distinctions like understanding and explaining. In everyday life mutual understanding occurs effortlessly, before theory or reflection; disturbance of it first startles us and makes us wonder. Communication with someone of alien origin, who speaks another language and who differs in mores and habits, requires a special effort; still in roundabout ways we may achieve understanding. This "entanglement" (Schapp) in our own situation does not entirely prevent us from entering into other environments. Even if we are not able to feel at home in them, we may well apprehend them in their peculiar character, distinguish them in their diversity, and relate them by contrast to our own. The breakdown of communication in psychosis however is more radical, more fundamental. Below the zero point of the norm monotony prevails. We do not deal with baroque or classicistic delusions or with ancient or modern, oriental or occidental schizophrenias. Whatever the language of the insane, the expressions of delusion are uniform. In the psychiatric clinic we discover the breakdown of mutual understanding in its elementary form beyond all historical variations. Psychiatry thus requires insight into the possibility of mutual understanding in its elementary structure, since it underlies all social and historical variants. Thereby it points to a philosophical problem which it cannot resolve by its own means. Psychiatry assigns to philosophy the task of revealing the axioms of everyday life and of making intelligible the possibility of communication. Thus we may finally be able to comprehend how far the eccentricities of our fellow man and his offenses against natural human orders, are to be understood as morbid, as manifestations of madness. During the ensuing dialogue between psychiatrist and philosopher the question will arise what significance philosophy attaches to clinical taxonomy with its distinction of organic, functional, and neurotic disorders.

To be sure, all attempts up until now to solve the problem of "intersubjectivity" by theories of analogical inference, empathy, inner perception, and appresentation, have failed, one after another. We are confronted with the amazing situation that what is obvious in everyday life, managed without difficulty by "kids" and grownups, by man and animal, defies all efforts to understand it in theory. This state of affairs strongly suggests that the question itself is unadmissible, and that the first thing to do is to pose the question correctly. In this regard psychiatric experience may be helpful.

Failure of communication remains in practice, though not always explicitly, the principal theme, the guiding motif [1]. Hallucinations can serve us for orientation here. A man complains that voices are insulting and threatening him or urging him to kill. He hears voices that we cannot hear. Since he is still speaking with us, communication with him is not entirely interrupted. Nevertheless mutual understanding is suspended. Someone might object that the patient hears better than we do. That one person hears or sees better than another is nothing unusual. Often the roles between doctor and patient are reversed. In an optometrical examination it is usually the physician who sees the test cards better, or at least knows them better than the examinee. The latter's mistakes in performance are interpreted as a minus, as a failure of his sensory apparatus, to be corrected with the help of instruments. The hallucinations, on the other hand, are not scored as a plus. We do not take the hallucinating patient to be divinely inspired. In setting ourselves up as judges and taking our own experience as the standard for the norm, we decide that he suffers from hallucinations. When I am alone with the patient, it is my conviction against his—one to

---

[1] Cf. RICHARD HÖNIGSWALD: Philosophie und Psychiatrie. Arch. Psychiat. 87, 715 (1929) as well as the papers by HENRI EY and MAURICE NATANSON in this book.

one. Still I anticipate that every normal person will confirm my judgment and not his. The patient, on the other hand, will not surrender his conviction, even though everyone else in the world should contradict him. Obviously this is a matter of diverse modes of being-in-the-world.

In everyday life one says that the patient hears something that is not real, something that does not exist. The psychiatrist agrees with the everyday view and defines hallucinations, for example, as "perception without object" [1]. This definition, which distinguishes two kinds of perception—those with and those without object—is based on a theoretical prejudice. The perceptions are conceived as mere subjective data of consciousness. Under normal conditions objects in the so-called external world are said to evoke subjective perceptions and to correspond with them in a certain way: in the case of hallucinations the "external stimuli" are said to be missing. Instead, the perceptual apparatus is supposed to be aroused by internal stimuli. Such retrogressive excitations are said also to evoke subjective images which, like all others, are projected "outwards". The hallucinative person, as psychoanalysis teaches in accordance with this fundamental thesis, withdraws from an intolerable reality, replacing it by a wish-fulfilling substitute.

LHERMITTE's definition is contradictory to both the experience of the everyday world and the clinic. To the patient the voices are by no means "subjective"; for him their reality is beyond doubt; the voices are objects of his pathological perception. So LHERMITTE's definition should read: hallucinations are perceptions without a common object. The tacit assumption is that the real world of visible and audible things is shared by us all. Withdrawal from reality signifies also for FREUD withdrawal from the reality that is essentially common. Unfortunately, this presupposition has not been expressed and critically examined. Instead it is emphatically rejected. This is unavoidable, since in such a theory perceptions are thought to be either physiological processes located in so many separate brains or sensory data distributed in this or that individual consciousness.

In normal circumstances an object is supposed to correspond to a perception. Even so, how could anyone, ensconced in the castle of his consciousness, a windowless monad, ever determine that "his" perception is in agreement with reality? If the "external world" were only accessible indirectly, by means of "reality testing", a process necessarily varying from individual to individual, how could an agreement between perception and reality ever be anticipated and attained? Under usual conditions one opinion would always be in opposition to another. The decision would have to rest with the majority. In actual fact just such an "operation" has been proposed as the solution to this problem. "Data are public", reads the formula, "when

---

[1] LHERMITTE, JEAN: Les hallucinations. Paris: Doin 1951.

shared by at least two observers". "... we may define objectivity as observational reliability ... each of at least two individuals has to do one observation per situational element. Objectivity is guaranteed when the observers agree ... Only such comparative oddities as, say, hallucinations, will spoil the ideal correlation [1]."

Such rules are extremely practical but also extremely naive. The stipulation of a majority being in agreement can of course reduce the errors in observation, but only with the additional conditions that the two observers work independently of each other, and be free from theoretical prejudices and disinterested with regard to the outcome. Lastly they must express themselves with perfect probity and derive identical meanings from their verbal exchanges. Shared observation points back to oral communication. With "verbalization" the initial difficulties then reappear. The requirement of a majority being in agreement is void; it will not guarantee objectivity, since it is applicable only under conditions that elude all objective observation. But this defect is still not the essential flaw. The crucial question, how it is possible that two observers view the same event together, has not only not been answered, it has not even been raised. A pair of observers are two, i. e. one plus another one, only from the standpoint of a third. Only he can compose the protocol statements made by one plus another one into a unity of two speakers and two reports. In their immediate relation to one another the observers are not two, one and one, but are related one to the other, for or against. Ordinarily we use cardinal numbers like adjectives; we speak of two observers—James and Jones—as under other conditions we speak of American scientists—Miller and Smith, or German scientists—Müller and Schmitt. In so doing we must guard against semantic misunderstanding. The adjectives "German" or "American" denote characteristics that apply to Miller as well as Smith, to Müller as well as Schmitt. Miller remains an American scientist, even without Smith, Müller a German scientist even without Schmitt. In the pair "James and Jones" each individual is one; they are two only as members of a group, but not in such a way that their separateness, one and another one, disappears in the group. What is remarkable about a common observation is just this, that two individuals, persons separate in their perceptions and as bodies, brains, and consciousnesses, are nevertheless able to observe one and the same event and to compare their findings.

In their immediate relation they stand vis-a-vis each other; they do not fuse. In a common observation the relation of the observers is not symmetrical. A common observation occurs in two phases: separate acts of observation, followed by a mutual exchange of statements. I compare what I see

---

[1] BRUNSWIK, EGON: The conceptual framework of psychology. Chicago: University of Chicago Press 1952, p. 11.

(or saw) with my own eyes with what the other tells me he has seen. Even with complete agreement our findings can never be made to coincide perfectly. The visible is one; our views are two and remain so. For communication there is no analogy in the physical or biological domains. In communication the separateness is at the same time both preserved and surpassed. That the visible is accessible to us all in common—the visible taken as a prototype—is the phenomenon enabling communication. Its power manifests itself in the fact that it never becomes a problem for us in everyday life. The very presence of the visible object is so compelling that it hides from us the separateness of the views. In actual fact, however, the other, my partner, together with whom I observe something, belongs to *my* visible surroundings. For me he is a visible object, just like the chair on which he is sitting. Of course I grasp this "object" as an experiencing being, who is able to direct himself like me and with me to the visible. The unification of our views of what is seen with our statements about it is nevertheless effected singly by the one or the other of us, even when *we,* in reciprocity and solidarity, find ourselves members of a *We.* No one else can perform the seeing of the visible for me, any more than he can assume my breathing and eating, waking and sleeping, living and dying. Someone else can relieve me at an observation post; he can continue the observation I have begun, but not my act of observing.

In science as well as in everyday life the visible is taken for granted. Physiological optics establishes itself in the domain of the visible, without making visibility a problem. It studies the eye as an optical instrument in relation to physically reduced light. It fails to consider the relation of the see-r to the see-able, although its experiments presuppose that experimental subjects and experimental devices are visible to the experimenter himself and that he is able to direct himself, together with the experimental subject, to something visible to both of them.

It may be useful to elaborate on the obvious with one more example. Say that I am in a museum, lost in the contemplation of a painting. Another visitor comes up from behind me, at first unnoticed. His mere presence doesn't affect my view of the picture; it neither adds nor takes anything away. Now that he has moved forward several steps, I notice his presence; even so my view of the painting remains as it was before. Looking straight ahead I face the picture; twisting around I see the other visitor and understand him as someone inspecting the same object. While the rays reflected from the picture plane, the stimuli, diverge in separate bundles to his eye and to mine, our gazes converge on the same object. If he should open a conversation and point something out to me that had previously escaped my notice, then I discover something in the see-able that he has already seen for himself. I cannot participate in his seeing; it is forever inaccessible to me. But I can, through his guidance, make actually accessible to my own view something that in principle is visible to both of us. Between me—the one looking-in-seeing—and him—the one-seen-looking—the spoken word mediates, which, as audible sound, is intelligible to the speaker and to the listener alike. In our conversation we both use the pronouns "I" and "you", though in reversed meaning. I well understand that when he says "I" he means himself, just as I refer to myself when I use the word "I". In our conversation *about* a visible object we speak with one another facing each other. If I wish once more to apprehend the object of our discussion visually, the initial situation is at once reconstituted.

Communication is mediated in the last analysis by the sensible. No intersubjective bridge links one wordless monad with another. Communication cannot be solipsistic, though it is, to be sure, egocentric, so that the other, seen from my position, is a part of the world opened to me, the world into which I find myself inserted as a part. Communication is im-part-ing; I meet the other one as a part-ner.

We view communication as a fact and as beyond any doubt; only the what and how require discussion. This attitude can be justified by pointing out that every discussion, pro and con, is conducted in human language, so that the fact is silently acknowledged as a fact from the very start, even if the discussion should end in a vociferous disagreement. We do not postulate an isolated, encapsulated consciousness as primary; we do not begin with the assumption of a solitary, empirical, or even transcendental, ego, only to wonder afterwards how such a monad could possibly arrive at the comprehension of an alter ego. Nor are we satisfied with the ontological reference to a "Being-with", which would call necessarily for a correlative "Being-separate". We consider communication as a mundane event, and shall attempt to encompass the role of the visible as mediator in a comprehensive fashion. Though the role of mediation is not confined exclusively to the visible, it certainly is eminent, and in a way that is different from the other modes of sense experience within which communication primarily occurs.

III. The Relation to the Allon

1. *The Visible as the Third and as the Other*

What is visible to you and me in common is, in relation to us both, a Third, and in relation to each one of us, the Other. That must be so, for only a Third, accessible to you as well as to me, yet nevertheless distinct from you and me, can remain vis-a-vis us both and can be shared by us. The visible can be a Third for us only when it is the Other in its respective relationships to me and to you [1]. We, you and I, do not encounter one another in a void; we do not confront one another immediately as ego and alter ego. Therefore a discussion of my relation to the Allon, which mediates between us, must accompany if not precede a discussion of our communicative relationship.

The visible does not belong to me like body and my limbs, like my pain and my pleasure, nor even like my thoughts, memories, or expectations. I can't read your thoughts; mine I can hide. You can't rummage around in my memories but have to wait until I tell you about them, i. e. express them in words audible to both of us. From my reports others are able to become acquainted with my life history, but even then my memories do not become theirs. In talking I can always keep my real opinion to myself or even attempt to mislead another. If he "speaks from the bottom of his heart", his complaints may stir me; this will happen if I take a friendly interest in him—but it doesn't have to happen. In a facing of the visible, however, there are no distinctions of rank or person, friend or foe. The visible is open to all alike. True, we can also hide a visible thing, but only behind other visible things. What is hidden is then excluded from my sight as well as from his; the visible appears or disappears for everyone at the same time; the sun shines alike on the just and the unjust.

For centuries the view has been held—as it still is today—that memories and phantasy images are decayed (HOBBES) or faded (HUME) sensations or that they are reactivated engrams (SEMON), which the sense stimulus has engraved into the plastic network of nerves. If this were so, then it should be expected that under special circumstances the faded ideas would re-acquire their original freshness. Such an assumption actually underlies most of the currently accepted theories of hallucinations and dreams. But no power in the whole world can make my phantasy images visible to another. The torch of a dream shines for no one else.

The subjectivistic interpretation of perception, dating back to GALILEO, reinterprets the actual relation of the see-r to the see-able as an appearance of perceptual images in a consciousness, thereby ignoring a fundamental characteristic of sensing and perceiving: the possibility of shared experience. A perceptual image "in me" cannot be simultaneously an object "in the external world", certainly not the object of common sight. Sensory data cannot face me, cannot look at me. A dogma blocks understanding, prohibits recognition even of the commonplace truths of everyday life. Cities and streets, temples and churches, courthouses and theaters have from time immemorial all been built with the unchallenged conviction of the possibility of a common view. The enormous assembly places of ancient and modern times demonstrate what happens everywhere every day.

---

[1] The Other here does not denote this or that fellow man, this or that particular thing. To avoid confusion, I will henceforth use the expression "the Allon".

In the modern Olympic stadium tens of thousands watch a race visible to all of them at the same time. When the decisive moment draws near, everyone feels *his* own heart beat, although the event that makes the particular spectator hold his breath is not his. The arena, the start and finish, sport and victory, are, in relation to each spectator, a part of the Allon; nevertheless for all of them they are one and the same. There, at the goal that all can see, this moment is shared by all; the contest has just been decided. At the day's end the throngs return home, each person aware of having witnessed a single great event entered in sports annals as an Olympic record. And those who have been there will be able to tell about it wherever and whenever they wish.

The visible and the seen are the same for all, despite the striking dissimilarity of views. In a theater one axis dominates: audience—stage. In a stadium on the contrary, where seats are placed toward all directions of the compass, views intersect. Despite such enormous differences which can easily be documented photographically, all present see the same arena and the same contests. Nor should it be forgotten that at a small board black and white play the same game from opposite positions.

In these changing views the visible never presents itself completely, although intended in its own order and totality. In relation to the visible we understand our own views as particular and variable, as positions which can be improved by changing our seats or coming nearer. The relation to the Allon, present even for someone who is the sole spectator in the huge oval of a stadium, provides access to it for others. There can be a public only where individuals find themselves ordered into a whole that encompasses them as its parts. If one could mark the directions of the spectator's gazes by threads, they would all converge on the same spot in the arena. This locus, appearing in a different perspective from each position, is, as a place *there*, necessarily relative to the *here* of each particular spectator. So while it is true that the *thither* goal enters into manifold relationships, it is not determined by them. The spectators direct themselves to a goal whose position has been fixed by its relationship to other places in the spatial whole of the arena, just as it could be determined by a surveyor. The perspective views are oriented toward a geometrical or, in any event, geometrically determinable "objective" order, invariant, valid, and binding for all.

In everyday life we move around in the never-to-be-doubted conviction that all spatial loci are particular ones, i. e., belonging to the single space continuum. Within this whole also our own place is determinable in relation to and reversion from others. We see in perspective, but the perspectives are transparent to us with regard to the order of things (of the Allon) as manifested in the various constancy phenomena. This was one of the factors that delayed the discovery of the laws of perspective in European painting.

Common sense does not suffice to elucidate the achievements of common sense. Perspective representation in painting soon resulted in the mistaken view that perspective vision also could be grasped entirely in a geometrical-optical fashion. In DÜRER's "Treatise" the eye (one eye) is represented as a focus towards which the light rays converge and from which the visual rays correspondingly spread out. The one who sees is inserted into space as seen, along with other things; the here and the there are treated as corresponding points in a geometrical network of relationships. The retina, in sensory physiology, is justifiably conceived as the end station for light falling upon it from the senders [1]. This terminal is then unjustifiably interpreted as the point of origin of the gaze. The "there" of the one who sees is, in dioptrics, constructed according to the same principles as the "there" of the seen. And yet the eye does not see itself; *the here is not seen at all.* The here is the "blind spot" in the total panorama. Whatever it may be that we see we look out at it "from here"; the place from which we direct ourselves towards other persons or things is determined by our relation to the ground, through "heft". The here of the person who sees is not an optical datum at all. The here, in opposition to the there, is my here. The visible, on the contrary, is, as mentioned above, not mine.

For me the visible is the other with which I am connected in a certain way but without being united with it. The relationship of "together in contraposition", a relationship that does not eliminate the separation but rather enhances it, characterizes all objectivity. As soon as I am no longer separate as a body subject, as soon as my relation with the Allon ends, so too does the community between you and me. We can admire together a bowl of delicious fruit arranged as a still-life but not the fruits we consume. That the "brutal" act of incorporation can decisively alter the relationship with the Allon makes it clear that this relation must be fundamentally one of the lived body. Since we are bound together in being separate, the together in contraposition implies freedom of movement. The relationship between the see-r and the seen cannot be that of a tightly fitted joint. In other words, only a motile creature, man or animal, can grasp the visible in its objective presence.

In everyday life we are rarely concerned with the relation of the person who sees to what is seen. Trusting that we are able to see things as they actually are, we turn our interest to the things seen and to their mutual relationships. These causal relationships have been carried over by the scientist

---

[1] Cf. BERKELEY's familiar argument, which touched off the centuries-old controversy about depth perception. "It is, I think, agreed by all, that distance of itself and immediately cannot be seen. For instance, being a line, directed end-wise to the eye, it projects only one point in the quick of the eye, which remains invariably the same, whether the distance be longer or shorter." (Essay Towards a New Theory of Vision.)

to the relation of the person who sees to what is seen. Sensory physiology equates this relation with that of a receptor to a sender. It reduces the one who sees to a sensory apparatus, which experiences certain effects from other bodies. The relationship with the Allon is thereby lost; for retina and brain, sensory data and perceptual images have no relation to the other as the other.

Since the visible shows itself to all of us together, it cannot be identical with stimuli, afferent impulses, or cortical excitations. Such events occur only *within* single organisms. They cannot be made congruent, even if there were something like an external projection of sensory data. The projections of my neighbor are not accessible to me, if only for the reason that in accordance with the theory my neighbor exists for me only as my projection. But the intentional objects of my solipsistic consciousness are just as unable to arise in another consciousness. The visible is not the intentional object of my consciousness, but it is truly an intentional object for me as a seeing, bodied being.

The visible does not appear to us within an "external world". The visible and I belong to one world, *the* world. I belong to the world, not the world to me. My egocentric encounter with the other takes place within the world common to all of us. We meet one another, as part-ners within *the* world, not in my world.

There seem to be good reasons for not viewing the relation to the visible and the possibility of mutual understanding as exclusively human privileges. In everyday life, anyone who feeds his dog is certain that the morsel he holds up is visible to them both, even if not in exactly the same way to the dog as to himself. Mutual understanding is not confined to the relationship between man and man. Its boundaries are more extended. There is a kind of mutual understanding between man and animal and animal and man and between animals. This fact is uncomfortable for every theory postulating an "analogical" understanding of the alter ego; nevertheless the fact still remains and demands consideration. Thus I do not think it appropriate to use the beautiful expression of "Being-in-the-world" in this context, since in HEIDEGGER's work it is understood as *existentiale*.

Communication requires the separateness of those who arrive at an understanding just as it requires something shared to mediate the mutual understanding. The fact of mutual understanding implies spatial distance between me and you and, likewise, spatial distance from such and such a mediating visible thing. Distance between me and you antecedes our mutual understanding; it does not vanish with understanding accomplished. The possibility of grasping separateness—a separateness that nevertheless permits union—is no less important for understanding communication than detecting the ways and means of con-vening. Every attempt to solve the problem of communication is predetermined by the interpretation of the separation to be bridged in reaching an understanding. From a radical separation in the "primordial" solitude of one's own life stream (HUSSERL), there is no access to "the other" within a world common to all of us. The meaning of "mime", of "my" lived body and also of "my" experiences is not given prior to any experiencing of the world. The meaning of "mine" is determined in relation to, in contraposition to, the world, the Allon, to which I am nevertheless a party. The meaning of "mine" is not comprehensible in the unmediated antithesis of I and not-I, own and strange, subject and object, constituting I and constituted world. Everything points to the fact that separateness and union originate in the same ground.

2. The Visible is Ruling

If the foregoing were not so, our highways would be littered with corpses. The drivers on a super-highway guide themselves in accordance with the structure of the road, despite differences of age and sex and of experience and skill. From his own position each grasps the same visible formation, the road and the cars that travel ahead of or toward him. Everyone is also aware of his own relationship to the street as stationary and to the vehicles as in motion. In seeing the visible he apprehends not only the surroundings, but simultaneously himself as the person who sees in his relation to what is seen. To be sure, he doesn't see himself, but even so his total experience reaches well beyond what is seen. This is ob-ject (Gegen-stand) for the one who in his selfhood (Selbst-ständigkeit) sees. The stimulus configurations do not correspond to the uniform apprehension of the visible.

The drivers who move from north to south, those who move in the opposite direction, and those on foot who cross the road at right angles, all of them grasp the road and their own positions in perspectives while oriented to the identical order of visible things in their own order. They see the identical but not the same. Somewhere WOELFFLIN tells the story of three young painters who planned to make an exact copy of the same landscape. When they compared their efforts, they discovered three drawings so different in style and conception that it was not easy to recognize the original they had in common. We might guess that the differences would be neither less nor more than the same words and sentences reproduced in three distinctive handwritings. We can be sure that one did not produce a mountain landscape, another a seascape, and the third a village street. Despite disparity of conceptions the visible prevails. CANALETTO and GUARDI saw Venice with different eyes; yet, although they painted Venice differently, they didn't paint a different Venice. It is easy to recognize the churches and palaces in the municipal portraits of both painters.

The visible both enables us to see it and demands of us that it be seen in a definite fashion. In every test of vision it is taken for granted that the

charts are visible in the same way to all. We expect the cooperative testee
to fulfill the demands inherent in each test chart. Of course he must assume
the right position; he must not turn his back to the charts; that's obvious
enough, but its full importance is not always realized. One need only
compare the behavior of the examiner with that of the testee. The examiner,
who knows the charts "by heart", carries his knowledge with him and can
use it at any time, wherever he goes, and in any position. What is remembered in remembering, what is imagined in imagining, is singularly
weightless. One who knows is related to things differently from one who
sees, for the visible is rendered accessible as definite and unique only in
actually turning toward it. We must come to meet the visible in order to be
affected by it. In order to see I must betake myself thence where the visible
shows itself, whereas the audible resounds. What is momentarily visible
shows itself as a section within a horizon of other possibilities toward which
one might direct oneself. The sight of the particular is embedded within the
context of our orientation in the field of gravity. Thus visible things themselves acquire for us their own "importance". In seeing we not only grasp
the visible but at the same time are aware of ourselves in our presence
(Dasein) as lived bodies in a relation to the Allon that is differently in-
flected in each sense modality.

Nevertheless the rule of the visible is not compulsory. The Allon
appears, as the examples make evident, in perspectives alone, and thereby
only in fragments, whose co-ordination is left to us. The "what" is never
given in its entirety. Every perspective reveals, but at the same time conceals, the structure of the Allon. It remains for each person to grasp the
structures of the visible from changing perspectives so that the fragments,
in their temporal sequence, can be brought into a meaningful order, into
which we also fit ourselves, i. e. into an order encompassing us all together.

The visible also prevails insofar as it is, or can be, the permanent, in
which we discover an abode. To the visible we can return and re-view it.
While the views are separated in a temporal succession the visible remains
identical. In the "firmness" of heaven, the firma-ment, as it was once the
custom to say, and on the "terra firma" the visible abides. It is such
reliability that accounts for the superior status of the present-at-hand in the
ontological tradition. For only the durability of the visible makes it
possible for us to act. The visible enables us and requires us to experience
it in a certain mode that holds for all.

3. The Visible is Encompassing

The expression "encompassing" is to be taken literally. It refers to a
mundane phenomenon, familiar to us in every daily situation. Whether we
stay within our four walls or venture outside, whether we enter our house

or step into the open under the spreading sky, we are always embraced by a horizon. Reference to a sur-rounding for man and animals points to the amazing fact that reaching beyond the boundaries of our own bodily existence we can com-prehend the encompassing as such and within it our-selves in relation to it. High, wide, deep, these words all refer to visible space as it opens itself to our gaze. An "apparatus" within the dimensions of the eye makes it possible for the person who sees to visualize spatial structures in the order of the magnitude of the surroundings. No other optical instru-ment can claim a comparable performance. A wide-open landscape or a gigantic building can of course be reproduced on a postcard, thus reducing the magnitude of the original to a tiny fraction. But the photograph itself does not see any other objects; nor does it comprehend its own magnitude relative to that of the building; it loses completely any compelling topical reference to the original, which lasted only for the moment of the film's exposure. The developed photograph does not look up to the original; its position in space makes no difference. It can be reproduced, and copies transmitted to all the countries of the world, to present the viewers with a picture of, say, the cathedral at Cologne. In the act of seeing, however, we see the cathedral or the mountain rises up before us, giants confronting a pygmy. But the pygmy is able to see the giant as such, the part is able to see the whole, the embraced the embracing, and to understand it in a certain way. If we go into the cathedral and let our eyes ascend the lofty pillars to the arches of the ceiling, or move along the nave to the altar and choir, then we realize how space expands out from us and ahead of us in many directions. In a picture drawn correctly in perspective, however, space contracts with the parallel lines converging to a vanishing point and the correctness of the perspective may be demonstrated scientifically. Space it seems either expands or contracts for the person who sees; but both cannot be true at the same time. And yet!—looking through the window I see vineyards on the other side of the valley rising way up to the horizon. If I take the window frames as my "frame of reference" then I can easily realize that the mountains, as seen at this moment, do not even occupy the whole window. In such a procedure the window has, of course, been used as the plane of projection. The hills are "brought forward" along the lines of vision and projected onto this plane. Thus we obtain a *picture*, which, to be sure, is differentiated into foreground and background, but one with-out any articulation into "here" and "there". It is a picture I contemplate, there in front of me, a picture cut out from the continuity of "real space" by a frame, a picture into whose proper space I cannot enter. The land-scape that I perceive is not, on the contrary, an image located in my con-sciousness.

The broad horizon of a landscape, the proportions of an architectural structure, help us to show the phenomenon of the encompassing. Yet the size of a visible object is not crucial. A stamp that two collectors inspect together is also a part of that space which encompasses both of them together. In relation to the horizon of everything visible the stamp appears small to us. There it can change places and pass from hand to hand. The stamp, separated from everything else by distinct boundaries, thus is surrounded by things that for the moment pass unnoticed. The particular is never given in radical singularity. As "something" it is forever related to something else from which it differs. All determination occurs in descent from an encompassing whole.

Seeing requires light. Reflected from things, it penetrates the eye, where, arousing the photosensitive elements of the retina, it becomes a stimulus. The visible objects do not go along with it. The Cologne cathedral is not absorbed materially by the observer, as the light is by the receptor. We see the cathedral in its immensity, in its form, and in its suchness—as *eidos* without *hyle*, to use the words of ARISTOTLE. It is enormous not in terms of a linear standard, nor even in comparison with the neighboring houses; it is tall in relation to ourselves. We see the facade towering up there before us in a common space and field of gravity. In our seeing we experience the real being-together of the visible and ourselves. Thus the *eidos* does not exclude substantiality, the burden of weight, solidity. We are not amazed that we can enter the cathedral through its portals, that it is worked on with hammer and chisel, that we are able to see it from all sides. To be sure, the "immateriality" of the relationship of the one who sees to what is seen resulted in the familiar misconceptions of "perceptual images" and "representations". This is not the place for a critical treatment of this tragedy of errors. It is evident, in any event, that a mere perceptual image must lack any relationship to the Allon. Just as a stimulus is received by a receptor, so supposedly the perception would be received by consciousness. From this solitary confinement there would be no egress. In the so-called perceptual images the visible has become invisible, at least for every other individual.

Common vision of the visible requires synchronization in the relation of those who come together. In communication my Now is encompassed by a moment of world time. The phenomenon of seeing and the relationship of the see-r to what can be seen are not derivable from the stimulus. Into the stream of stimuli one cannot descend a second time; stimuli must be constantly renewed. And yet we, together, are able to see objects and to see them again together or as individuals.

The relation to the Allon is not easy to grasp, for it is neither a relationship of two bodies nor of two souls; the familiar categories of cause and effect do not apply. The relation to the Allon is not calculable nor is it statable in equations. Its distinguishing feature is the inequality and not the equality of the relata.

IV. The Significance of Motility

Our relation to the Allon is a dialectical one, a contraposition or connection in separation. The visible does not belong to an external world from which we are separated by an impassable gulf. Everyday life knows nothing of the "primal splitting" (N. Hartmann) between see-r and seen, knower and known, which has kept metaphysics and epistemology going. Philosophy tends to reject the position of everyday life as naive realism; but the claims of the latter may be better grounded than skeptics are willing to admit. Turning aside from the "axioms of everyday life" (Erwin Straus), science has replaced "the interpretation of Dasein in its every-dayness" (Heidegger) by abstract constructs which nevertheless cannot completely be detached from the "life world" (Husserl) [1]. Naive realism, it seems, is born anew in every generation. Its adherents far exceed those of all other philosophical schools and this even without any proselytizing or teaching. In the naive realism of everyday life, the living reach an understanding among themselves and an understanding of the evidences of the past. The relation to the Allon and the belonging in contraposition manifest themselves powerfully in every consideration of the "objectivity" that guides the attitude of everyday life today as always: Things show themselves to us just as they are; the belong to us and yet are separated from us. Our gaze reaches them without changing them—action without reaction. We experience things as the object of our gaze, not as the cause of our seeing.

Natural realism refers back to human nature. The "scandal of philosophy" mentioned by Kant, namely its inability "to be able to bring any adequate proof for the existence of things outside ourselves", does not disturb the *life world*. In it, primordial divisiveness is paired with primordial solidarity. The *life world* is not an external world. The opposition to the Allon is based on a prior co-presence. How is it possible to comprehend this dialectical relation within mundane observation?

Heaven and earth were created before man. According to the Biblical account, the creation of man was God's last act of creation, the crowning deed of the entire work of creation. Man, who is said to have been created in the image of God and set to rule over the earth, remains an earthly creature. "Fish and fowl" were called into life on the fifth day; but "the beast of the earth, after his kind, and cattle after their kind, and every thing that creepeth upon the earth", they all were the work of the sixth day

---

[1] Husserl's term "Lebenswelt" refers to the every-day world but emphasizes its covert riches rather than its overt triteness. Therefore the literal, although cumbersome, translation "life world" is used.

preceding the creation of man. Just as animals were created as members
of a genus, each according to its kind, so too was the human being. "And
God created *man* in his own image ... male and female created he *them*."
The same verse that establishes the "unique place of man in the cosmos"
(SCHELER) emphasizes, in terms of genus and sex, the distance from the
creator, i. e. the animal nature of man. That he belongs to earth is even
more sharply expressed in the second story of creation: "And the Lord God
formed man of the dust of the ground". Both believers and unbelievers can
accept this natural determination of man's fundamental character insofar as
it merely says that man is an earthly creature, unexceptional in terms of his
material elements, and in a material community with all the earth through
his metabolism. There is also general agreement that man has been *made*
from the dust of the ground, i. e. formed into an individual organism.
Whether man, as the Bible states, owes his life to a creative act of God's in
which God's breath has been entrusted to him, or whether, as science teaches,
he has developed from other species in the course of a long evolution, it is still
a fact that he is a living being, a *zoon*, able to lift himself from the earth,
above the earth of which he is made. "For dust thou art and unto dust shalt
thou return"—between that beginning and that end earthly life takes its
distinctive course. The material kinship with earth does not exhaust the
relation of man and animal to earth.

Man and animal are so made or at least so organized that they are
able to get up from the supporting ground as motile beings and to oppose
themselves to it as individuals in self-af-firma-tion. We belong to the world
and yet stand opposite to it in singularity. The dialectical relationship of
togetherness in contraposition is grounded in motility. With it the primary
animal situation is given. Motility or living movement is the distinguishing
mark of man and animal. In regard to the meaning of "self-movement"
opinions differ widely; no one will deny, however, that for animal existence
the imperative holds: "Get up or die!" Getting up from the ground, over-
coming gravity, is basic for every active movement.

Getting up—"uprising"—precedes every partial or complete locomotion. The upward direction of plants is realized according to different
architectonic principles, as it were. The upward development against
gravity corresponds to the downward extension of the roots. Trees grow
upward, they don't stand up. The lower parts support the higher ones and
thrust them ahead of themselves. The crown of a tree cannot of its own
accord return to the ground; it cannot lie down. Man and animal, on the
contrary, rise up against gravity by means of their own strength; the
upright posture of man and terrestrial animals requires constantly renewed
effort. The lower part is no less sustained by the upper than the upper is
upheld by the lower. Gravity certainly is overcome in a particular manner,
but neither man nor animal is able to overcome it completely.

Standing up against the ground and locomotion are not merely two different forms of movement. If we consider the functions of muscles, joints, and nervous system physiologically, we find that in both standing up and moving forward, special mechanisms, similar in principle, enter into play. Yet standing up and locomotion are different when considered as modes of the relationship of the organism to the world.

Human movement from one place to another one can, in certain banal situations, be stated and demonstrated in terms of a mechanical scheme of movement. One can ascribe to it a beginning and an end. In locomotion we leave A behind spatially and temporally, and we arrive at B where for the time being we rest. In such a movement we reach a position determined as one single point within the surroundings. None of this applies to getting up. In getting up each one reaches a position counter to the world, entering into a *universal* contraposition tied to no one particular spot. In getting up we don't leave our place; it is just the Here which is constituted. In getting up we are not directed toward another spot, an inviting goal where we will be able to rest, as we are in moving from one place to another. Rather getting up requires constant effort in order to hold oneself upright. It implies the possibility of falling. In everyday life an order to take a rest is naturally understood as invitation to lie or sit down and thus as a transition to a position in which we no longer resist gravity. In the physical interpretation of movement bodily rest is described quantitatively as an equilibrium in the play of opposing forces, and descriptively as an event whose magnitude of movement approaches zero. Existence (Dasein) as lived body is ruled, quite differently, by the qualitative opposition of repose and exertion.

Getting up against gravity evokes heaviness ("heft") as a counterforce. In lifting ourselves from the ground we discover that we are held down, if not attached, to it. With every movement from one place to another the "here" migrates. But in getting up, in lifting ourselves above the ground while remaining bound to it, relationships to a visible "there" open themselves before us. So it is when we get up that the "contraposition in togetherness" is originally achieved. We can act in relation to something only insofar as we are able to comport ourselves in opposition to it. Comportment demands open possibilities, and these we are first given in getting up with its ever-present countermovement.

The difference between locomotion and getting up manifests itself in their differing accessibility to representation. Locomotion may be adequately represented—so at least it appears—in a schematic fashion, while getting up doesn't allow such a representation. Consequently movement from one place to another has become the model for the modern mathematical definition of physical movement as Descartes initially formulated it, namely: "displacement of a portion of matter or of a body from the proximity of bodies in immediate contact with it, and which we view as being at rest, into proximity with others" [1]. Descartes emphasized that by movement he simply understood movement from one place to another, "for I cannot imagine any other kind and I am of the view that we ought not to assume any other in nature".

It is easy to depict Descartes' definition of movement in a horizontal schema. If one adds to it a time line and a scale, then one can also read off the speed of the movement by which a body X is brought from the proximity of point A into that of point B. The body X could also be that of a human being who goes, or more precisely, has gone from A to B. There are still several devices, however, hidden within this simple, so easily understood schema. The diagram replaces the movement with its trajectory. In the schema we see start and goal simultaneously in *one* glance while we understand them as the point of departure and the terminal point of a single movement. Consequently the being-in-movement is not actually reproduced in such a comprehension; the movement is merely projected in a certain way onto a frame of reference that is at rest. We can do this because we are already "in the picture" in our original everyday observation of movement. We com-prehend what comes first and what follows in a manner that does not hold for the moved body itself. Actually in such a schema the motion, still incompleted, is represented as complete. In the simultaneous representation of A and B, the start and goal, as experienced, say, by runners in a race, are not considered at all. Only a few isolated parameters of the happening are reproduced. The schematic representation that permits mathematical treatment is a most inadequate rendering of the phenomenon, since the segment A-B is to be understood as a continuum of infinitely numerous divisible parts and correspondingly the movement of body X as a passage through a continuum of infinitely many phases. But intended movement is directed beyond the distance itself, toward a goal "still not" reached and is an action performed literally, in many separate steps. To those who tried to escape from East Berlin, for example, A and B were by no means indifferent and simultaneously given points. From B, a place that they saw before them, but had not yet reached, from this already visible and yet still remote goal, safety beckoned. The passage from A to B was a mortal avenue; in leaving A they did not know whether it would be granted them to reach B. Yet in this unique race with death it is only the habitual situation of man and animal that is thrown into relief. By nature man and animal are compelled to seek their nourishment, their own kind, and shelter against heat and cold. Man and animal do not move in mathematically homogeneous space. Locomotion is linked with terrestrial space, which opens up to the individual zones of what is desirable and what is to be avoided. Every intended

---

[1] Descartes: Principles of Philosophy. Pt. II, par. 20.

movement is aimed at "the better", not something higher or better as enjoined by an ethical code, but something actually desired, something that appears preferable to the individual at a given moment. Self-movement is not distinguished from other forms of movement by a particular releasing device or by particular mechanisms of performance; self-movement is intelligible only as comportment towards the world, as an I-world relation.

Because of their antinomic structure, rising up and standing upright resist schematic formalization. By analogy to the horizontal schema of movement from one place to another one might consider representing rising up by means of an additional vertical axis. But rising up is not a climbing movement that gradually and in time raises the body as a whole above the starting level to a higher spot. Rising up ends in standing upright—it ends so to speak in itself. We gain the "above" without losing the "below". When we are upright we still remain beneath. The grave and stately gait of a ceremonial march expresses both at the same time: being lifted above the ground and having a firm foothold on it.

Locomotion as human and animal movement, in accordance with the polar differentiation of the lived body, is normally directed forward. But the point of departure for one person is the target for another; in going to the station we meet others coming from it. Hither and thither, the directional meaning of (forward-aiming) locomotion relative to the surroundings are always individually conditioned by life history. But the "below" is universal, always the same for all; we never entirely escape from it. Standing up is the fundamental position, or, more correctly, in getting-up we secure the primary position, which, because of its ever-present tie with the countermovement, possesses the character of actuality, in its double sense of presence and comportment. Monumental art represents only the dead as recumbent.

In place-to-place movement a path is traced; for rising-up there is, to be sure, a technique, but no way. Thus, in a schema for locomotion one can represent the moved body by a symbol being displaced on a line from A to B. Such a representation is inadequate for rising up. An arrow would be a more suitable symbol since the arrow takes account of the polar differentiation of the body subject into head and feet. And yet to symbolize getting-up by rotating an arrow 90 degrees from the horizontal to the vertical would still be a questionable expedient. In getting up we not only turn the length-axis of our own body by a right angle, but enter into another relationship to the ground, namely that of the counter-position. As a rule we signify the unilateral direction "from—to" by an arrow; in getting up the direction upward (vertical-crownwards) is paired with the direction downwards (perpendicular). Therefore getting up cannot be represented by a curve marking the course of the center of gravity in getting up. For when the rotation of the length-axis has been completed the center of gravity is not upright. The relationship of "belonging in contraposition" is a *macro-scopic* relation, in which the microscopic structures as such do not participate.

We have all too long sought universal scientific salvation in analytic methods, in procedures that extend downward to the cells, cell parts, and molecules. The microscope is a marvelous instrument. The images of fibrils and filaments brought up from hidden depths with its help appear so valuable and amazing that we are inclined to forget the simple truth that the fibrils function meaningfully only within the macrostructure of muscles as each one of them has been designated by its own anatomical name. What occurs there at the level of molecules acquires meaning only by coordination with events on an entirely different level: that of the comportment of the organism towards its surroundings. The macroscopic relation cannot be derived from the microscopic states. The body is upright as a whole, not as bones, muscles, and cells. Neither tissue nor tissue parts, neither organ nor system, are in the relation of part to the whole of the world, of belonging in contraposition. The feet of the human being who stands upright are horizontal, while his arms hang down from his shoulders. The position of the "raised head" "depends" on the downward contraction of the neck and shoulder muscles. The mechanisms of movement within the organism and the position of the organism in the world vis-a-vis the world are not parallel. When we stretch our arm forward, sideward, or upward, then the contraction of the adductor and extensor muscles is directly contrary to the resulting movement of the arm and hand. There is no doubt that in standing up a relation to the ground is realized that exists for the animated and lived body as a whole, but not likewise for its parts. In getting up, man and animal achieve a position of their own, which is both a belonging-to, and a maintaining of, a contra-position. This is probably the root meaning of "ex-sistere", the one nearest to the sensorially most immediate event, namely, a standing up from that ground that sustains us. As motile beings we enter into opposition to the Allon, to which we never-theless remain bound. Primary separation is paired with primary solidarity. One relationship is not possible without the other. Separation—felt as such —calls for connection—realized as such. Only motile beings are able to be in a relation to the Allon or, stated differently, only for motile beings can there be sensory experience.

One could hardly claim that the traditional interpretation has recognized the fundamental importance of motility. That a body "moves by itself" is of course for us a practical sign that such a body is a living organism, man or animal. The motoric expressions, however, do not interest us here as a betokening of life; rather we want to emphasize that the power to rise from the ground and to oppose oneself to the ground is the indispensable condition for sensory experience. Only a creature capable of rising from the ground and thereby contraposing itself to things can establish sensory ties with them in the amphiboly of contact and distance. Consciousness is the natural privilege of motile creatures. This proposition is confirmed by the changes in behavior that occur in the daily alternation of waking and sleeping.

Everyone knows that the movement-apparatus, consisting of bones and muscles, forms the bulk of human and animal bodies. It is hardly a disputed fact that if consciousness exists at all, it does so only for motile creatures, and that their sensory experience of the world, alternating between sleep and waking, "arises" only when they do. Science possesses an extremely rich knowledge about the structure and arrangement of the movement-apparatus. But insight into the fundamental implication of rising against gravity—"fundamental" in the literal sense of the word—for human and animal experiences has not developed to the same degree.

"I have never seen nor understood", wrote DESCARTES, "that human bodies have consciousness, but only that it is the same humans who have consciousness *and* who have a body". To that view we oppose this proposition: only corporeal, motile beings can be endowed with consciousness. But didn't DESCARTES, and we with him, have good reason to wonder? Can that *and* be dismissed so lightly? This question may be countered with another one: is DESCARTES actually speaking, in agreement with his own presuppositions, of the human body and human consciousness? Philosophers, accepting DESCARTES' own interpretation, have understood his distinction of substances—as applied to man—as a radical separation of body and soul. Thus GILSON, for example, compares the Cartesian dichotomy with Aquinas' conception of the relation of body and soul. The body in DESCARTES' interpretation, however, is by no means identical with the body considered by AQUINAS. The *res extensa* is not body in everyday usage nor in medicine. DESCARTES actually wondered how empty geometrical space could be united with the abstract self-consciousness of the Cogito. This certainly is a perplexing problem—thwarting all efforts to find a solution. Instead of trying again, we will modify the question and ask how a body bound by gravity, a lump of clay, can transcend its own boundaries and grasp the world as Allon. Going beyond the empirical observation that only living beings like man and animals are bearers of consciousness—DESCARTES' "and"—we have tried to show that only motile beings are capable of experiencing; the relation, however, is not that of a carrier and the one carried, who from his vantage point inspects the world from above. In rising up from the ground man and animal achieve that contraposition to the world which rules the structure of all experiencing.

It is tempting to relate the devaluation of movement to the trend toward inwardness that began with AUGUSTINE. Yet it is to be recalled that it was precisely the subjectivism of GALILEO and DESCARTES that served them in founding modern natural sciences as a pure doctrine of movement.

DESCARTES, it is well known, assigned the movement of men and animals to the realm of inanimate bodies. Such a classification was an inevitable consequence of his metaphysics, from which radically new problems were encountered. One of them was how to understand the capacity of the human soul to intervene in bodily happenings. The other task, no less difficult, was to show how the apparently meaningful comportment of animals could be "re-duced" to meaningless mechanical events. Animal movement was not to be purposive, not goal-directed; it was not to be the action of an animal directing itself visually towards a distant object. DESCARTES discovered—or postulated, actually—the reflex, which enabled him to explain the comportment of an animal towards its surroundings as an event within the animal organism. Strictly as a consequence of his physical principles, long before empirical research, he reduced the movements of men and animals to microscopic events, to movements of the tiniest corpuscles (animal spirits) in the tubular system of the nerves that he hypothesized. Self-movement was unmasked as the movement of a marionette. Every meaningful comportment of an organism towards the world in its macroscopic order was annulled. As its correlate DESCARTES' mechanical explanation of movement required a similar mechanistic explanation of sensation. It was precisely the Cogito, leading to an interpretation of "external" sensations as purely subjective and confused ideas detached from the world, which also enabled DESCARTES to interpret the sensory process as one of motion, that is, of the "animal spirits". Thus man and animals no longer stand as individuals within the world opposite to it; they are to be investigated as particular bodily aggregates in the total field of physical events, a program to which objective psychology has devoted itself. Radical subjectivism thus ends up in radical objectivism.

The significance of motility for self-preservation has always been recognized. The significance of motility for consciousness still awaits recognition. Theologians and philosophers have readily attributed to the soul the faculties of perception and thought, phantasy and memory, feeling and desire. Even "specious" sensation has been admitted to the kingdom of reason; but movement has been exiled. Movement remains but a corporeal event even for those who teach that the soul, when desiring and willing, sets the body into motion. The soul does not climb trees or jump ditches; it does not bite and swallow, even when it is hungry and thirsty. Of course it is known that an animal must move to stay alive. But since animal movement can be meaningful only when it is directed by sensations, the status of sensation appears to be prior and superior to that of movement. Although in WEIZSÄCKER's doctrine of the "Gestalt circle" this subordination has been replaced by coordination, the general relation of sensorium and motorium has been interpreted as similar to that of an operator and his machine. An external contact with the surroundings is, then, apparently accomplished through the senses, but the movement still takes place *within* the organism. That is certainly one of the reasons why both sensualists and idealists were willing to accept sensations and perceptual "images" as contents of consciousness, while motor events were at most represented by goal images and kinaesthesias. "But intuition", says KANT, "takes place only insofar as the object is given to us. This again is only possible to man at least, insofar as the mind is affected in a certain way [1]." Just as here, in the first paragraph of the "Transcendental Aesthetics", reference is made to us humans, so at the outset of the following section, containing a "metaphysical exposition of the concept of space", it is said that "by means of outer sense, a property of the mind, we represent to ourselves objects as outside us, and all without exception in space" [2]. The "Critique of Pure Reason" thus proposes to start from the situation of man. But nowhere does that great work consider us humans as live-bodied, mobile beings. The connection with man is reduced to observation of the sensory sphere divorced from motility; simultaneously the sensory sphere is conceived as an organization, which transmits a manifold of world-free sensory data to higher "authorities" for synthesis. Although transcendental knowledge occupies itself "with our mode of knowing of objects, insofar as this is said to be possible apriori", KANT's criticism does not consider "our mode of knowing" with regard to man, but reconstructs it with regard to—or actually looking back from— mathematical physics. His transcendental aesthetics treats of space and time; of gravity and man's getting up from the ground that supports himself, there cannot be, in conformity with the whole orientation of his work, any mention. Man, whose mode of knowing is supposedly being investigated, is simply not inserted into earthly space as a live-bodied creature. The sensory sphere, affected by the objects, sits—so it appears—atop the mobile live body like a camera mounted on a dolly. A good-natured simpleton, the motor-apparatus carries the burden of reason without realizing—like the legendary Christopher—what it is upholding. It deserves no consideration and it receives none.

The dethronement of living movement had already begun of course in antiquity. In the Aristotelian hierarchy of living creatures it is the faculty of sensation (aisthesis), and not motility, which distinguishes animals as opposed to plants. "... it is the possession of sensation that leads us for the first time to speak of living things as animals [3]." ARISTOTLE expressly excludes observation of animal motion from his treatise "De Anima". In a later passage he explains in a more detailed way not only why *aisthesis*

---

[1] KANT: Critique of Pure Reason. (Norman Kemp Smith) London: Macmillan 1956, p. 65.

[2] KANT: Critique of Pure Reason. (Norman Kemp Smith) London: Macmillan 1956, p. 67.

[3] De Anima, 413 b, 2—4.

should occupy a privileged status, but also why motion does not present a *purely* psychological topic. The connection is this: bodily-movement is instigated by desire. But desire itself is elicited by what is desirable. "The instrument which appetite employs to produce movement is no longer psychical, but bodily [1]." Aristotle concludes the section of desire and movement in "De Anima" with the words: "Insofar as an animal is capable of desire it also possesses self-movement". He does not arrive at the contrary conclusion: that only a being capable of self-movement is able to direct itself—in longing—toward another *as other*.

ARISTOTLE conceived animal movement generally as loco-motion, as movement determined by its goal. Rising up does not take priority for him, because it is not initiated from elsewhere by something desirable. In getting up we seek nothing and accomplish nothing outside ourselves; nothing is aimed at save standing upright, which indeed opens up unlimited possibilities. In subsequent sections I will try to show how man's mode of placing himself into the world and of his standing bodily within it affect the total structure of his experience in times of health and illness.

V. The Primary Animal Situation

The act of getting up may be considered as upbeat for what is to come; yet it is far more than that. In getting up from the ground man and animal realize a relation to the world that we shall call the primary animal situation (animale Ursituation) [2]. In the primary situation we enter the realm of primary orientation, a realm we explored with the intention of satisfying vital needs. The Allon that we oppose in getting up presents the visage of Mother Earth who "bears us and cares for us": For She is just that other from which we stem and to which we belong. The Allon is both *hostis* and *hospes*, though at times the hospitality must be wrested from it. Manna fell from heaven only once.

When we get up, a tension arises between our slender basis and the surrounding vastness which at the same time attracts and deters. This contrast never vanishes completely; for the Here, no matter how far we stray, always comes along with us. The Here in which we take a firm stand detains us. With the wide spaces opened to us in getting up, we experience at the same time the weight of our confinement. Heaviness ties us to the

---

[1] De Anima, 433 b, 18—20. Ross, W. D.: Works of Aristotle. III. Oxford: Clarendon Press 1931.

[2] The upright posture of man is a unique case, which at this moment requires no special consideration. In order to avoid the continuous repetition: "man and animal", I will simply speak of "us" and "we". These personal pronouns will frequently refer also to the animals, as indicated by the context.

proximate and screens our fantasy from Faustian yearnings. Even when, self-detached, lost in thought, we do yield to our imagination, a sudden sound, a slight touch, a gleam of light, are enough to bring us back from our distraction into the present and set us right. Only in deep sleep do we elude the binding power of the Here.

Actually we should not refer to "we" and "us"; for the word "here" is a personal qualification; when it is detached from the speaker it loses any "tangible" meaning. We cannot date a letter with Here or Now; only in a second step do we determine the here as a place in geographical space and the now as a temporal point on the calendar. To answer the question "Where are we?" with "Here", would be, although correct, meaningless. For we, both questioner and answerer, are always somewhere Here. With the expression "here" I point to a place that I "occupy" in passing. In the actuality of pointing to it, my Here is inseparable from my Now. Here designates a place where I am staying right now—in contrast to many other possible locations. The word Here is one of the expressions HUSSERL called "occasional". They are called so because specific events determine their precise meaning. As mine, the Here is unequivocally determined by my presence, while in relation to the world, its meaning remains entirely equivocal. The Here that is unfailingly mine manifests my basic relationship with the world, which persists without modification as a conjunction in opposition.

The "my" is not a primary phenomenon of pure consciousness that precedes experience of the "real world", as taught by HUSSERL in his "Ideas I" and also in modified form in his posthumous published works. In his "Considerations on the constitution of the natural world in the absolute consciousness" [1], HUSSERL posed the question of how it is possible for "the absolute consciousness, so to speak, to come into the real world?"—"*Thus on the one hand consciousness should be the Absolute*, within which everything transcendent is constituted ... and on the other hand consciousness should be a subordinate real event within this world. How does this tally?" To illustrate the opposition, HUSSERL makes use of a radical phantasy reminiscent of DESCARTES: "Let us imagine ... that the whole of nature—and the physical in the first instance—has been 'annulled', so there would then be no more bodies and therefore no men. As a man I should no longer be, and again I should have no neighbors. But my [sic!] consciousness, however its states of experience might vary, would remain an absolute stream of experience with its own distinctive essence" [2]. The "my" appears here as a primordial datum. But it is incomprehensible how any meaning would accrue to "my" in the radical solitude of absolute consciousness. In a

---

[1] HUSSERL, E.: Ideas I. New York: Macmillan 1931, p. 164.
[2] HUSSERL, E.: Ideas I. New York: Macmillan 1931, p. 164.

magnificent shifting of fronts Husserl seeks to ground the "animalia and the psychological consciousness" in transcendental consciousness. In doing so, he obviously ascribes characteristics to absolute consciousness that have been borrowed from man as empirical subject. The original sense of "my" is comprehensible only as opposition—through the deed of self-assertion—against the Allon, which "edges near" to me or—seen from my point of view—which I contact. The "my", which is always implied in the "here", does not denote, first and foremost, what is mine, as a possession, or anything that belongs to me. Originally it denotes a relation to the world, in contrariety and attachment. In this relation the world does not appear as *my* world, but as the one encompassing world of which I am a part and within which, as a motile body subject, I can occupy now this place, now that. Individuation is a natural relation to the world; it is not grounded in the mineness of the Being of existence (Dasein), which comports itself towards its own Being [1]. The "I am" and "I do" express a relation to the world that is singular and unique for each speaker and yet generally valid for all.

With the possessive "my", as possession, I lay claim to something else as mine, which, however close it may be to me, is not yet one with me, whereas the "my" of the "here" is inscribed in my own body ("Leib"), so to speak, for in this instance I emerge as precisely the one who makes the claim. As such I stand within the solitude of my own bodily existence in the world yet vis-a-vis to it. That to which I lay claim, house and home, wife and child, belongs—like a neighbor and all that is his own—to the Allon. And yet my relation as a claimant to what is claimed is not that of subject to object, nor of an inner to an outer world.

The inventory of what is originally mine may be put in just these two words: bare life. This was the entire "belongings" that a Cynic philosopher named, according to tradition, as he jumped overboard from a sinking ship, crying, "Omnia mea mecum porto". Of course his belongings included senses and movement, thoughts and memories, speech and accomplishments.

The "my" of the lived body, its belonging to me and my belonging to it, is not a relation of possession. What belongs to me can be taken away from me by others; what I claim as a possession can be disputed by others; what I would like to have others can give to me. Others can mutilate or destroy my body, but they cannot give it to me. The possession of everything that I secondarily claim as "mine" is an enlargement of the original region of the Here, which in getting up I stake out in the Allon. Bare life already resides in the Allon. Within it there is a zone we make our own as a "possession" by setting up, visibly or invisibly, the "fence" Rousseau

---

[1] An allusion to Heidegger: "We are ourselves the entities to be analyzed. The Being of any such entity is *in each case mine*. These entities, in their Being, comport themselves toward their Being". Being and Time, p. 67.

mentioned, the fence that shuts out, or should shut out, everyone else. For just as I reach over into the Allon and isolate what is my own, so that which is most immediately my own is threatened by the invasion of the Allon. The stance of opposition to the Allon does not open up an unbridgeable chasm. Mine and Not-mine are divided by a boundary, which separates what originally belongs together.

The dual role of my own body corresponds to the conjunction in opposition that characterizes the relationship to the Allon. It is my own *lived* body, the body I am, but also the body I have[1]. HUSSERL tried to grasp this "dual aspect" in terms of the opposition of the inner kinesthesia to the externally real movements of the body[2]. Nevertheless the real bodily movements remain mine, even as "external" movements. In speaking, I both produce myself and hear my own voice. In a chorus I join my voice with other voices in a polyphonic symphony. My opposition to the world does not exclude me from the world. With my hand I take another's hand, feeling and answering to the clasp of his. I take a pen to write my letters and to sign them with *my* signature. I see myself in the mirror; I inspect my image reflectively and dress my own body to agree with aesthetic convention. But not only do I hear my voice and see my hand exactly as I see others' hands; I breathe, eat, and drink; I am in active exchange with the Allon. I take something of it into myself. Should we really believe that, in eating, a subject incorporates an object or that an object—the food—is carried in the proximity of another object with the support of still other objects, such as hands, forks, and spoons? The relationship to the Allon is not one of radical opposition nor one of a subject that perforce, in one leap, must transcend an abyss to the object beyond. Such an assumption is unavoidable only if one makes pure consciousness the subject of experience and action[3]. Man, who gets up from the ground, is never radically cut off from the Allon. Nonetheless the tension implied in the opposition of subject and object is not excluded from the relationship to the Allon. Indeed, the tension of opposition still exists, but only dialectically paired with attachment. All encounters on the whole scale from the polite greeting to the mutual embrace occur within the relationship to the Allon as the ground from which one's fellow man detaches himself as *heteros*. Thus the boundary towards the Allon is not a sharp divide, separating what is on this side from what is on that side so that "my own body" would be situated on this side and everything else on the other; nor does all bodily experience fit the one schema of dual aspects mentioned by HUSSERL. Here is a clinical example: anosognostic patients, i. e., persons

---

[1] Cf. JÜRG ZUTT: Auf dem Wege zu einer anthropologischen Psychiatrie. Berlin-Göttingen-Heidelberg: Springer 1963.

[2] Husserliana VI. S. 164. Haag: Martinus Nijhoff 1954.

[3] Cf. HEIDEGGER, M.: Being and Time, pp. 85—86 and passim.

stricken with hemiplegias—mostly left lateral ones—are unable to recognize by sight their motorically and sensorially paralyzed limbs as their own. It has been assumed that this paradoxical behavior expresses an unconscious denial of the defect. And yet my hand, for example, as seen does not differ in principle from other visible things, say, the top of the desk on which it rests. As a visible shape my hand has not been marked by a sign of ownership. A clever arrangement of mirrors might embarrass someone who had to decide whether a hand pointed at in a mirror among many others were his own or not. But at the very moment the finger is touched instead of being seen, every doubt evaporates. In every contact I feel myself touched, no matter whether I am touched on the hand, on the forehead, or on the back. The skin is not the outer surface of a body but the bounding plane of the body subject, which, like all boundaries, both separates and joins. When I move my hand actively and when I am touched on it then I originally experience my hand as mine. The "my" of the body subject is experienced in a distinctive manner in each sense modality. The tactile "my" is without an analogy in the optical sphere. We are able to sing in the dark, but we are unable to shine—unlike the firefly—at night. The *lumen naturale* that enabled man to make candles, lamps, and floodlights, does not illuminate "the palpable obscure". Pictures and mirrors lack any counterpart in the tactile sphere. I see my hand there, in the same place where I see the desk, paper, and pencil. Everything visible has the quality of "there". The "here", however, is not seen, but constitutes itself in the reciprocity of the immediate, motor, tactile contact. The impressions of touch are not integrated into an open horizon like those of vision. Only in the light can I see my hand; with darkness it is removed from sight and so becomes inaccessible to sight, just like my eyes and back. Darkness subtracts nothing, light adds nothing, to the immediate experiencing of my own body. The anosognostic patient, whose limbs are no longer at his disposal, is unable to recognize the paralyzed arm as his own merely by glancing at it. Occasionally one can demonstrate to such patients that the body part that appears strange to them must be their own. But such secondary insight is unable to prevail very long against the elemental force of sensory impression or, to be precise, of the void of sensory impression.

Since our relation to the world takes the form of contraposition, of dehiscence rather than a radical break, there is no radical separation of subject and object. Both, complete belonging and complete distance, suspend the relationship to the Allon. The Allon as such can never become entirely ours. The very moment we make a part of it ours, as in eating and drinking, or become wholly a part of it, as in falling asleep, it is no longer the Other. In the dialectic of accessibility and remoteness, of hiddenness and openness, the Allon remains enigmatic, either in its entirety, like the world that KAFKA put on trial, or as an individual person, like Desdemona, murdered by the doubting and despairing Othello. Jealousy is rooted in the insoluble duplicity of the Allon, whose taciturnity in one's encounter with another human being, the heteros, mounts to silence and reticence. Without the possibility of denying oneself the giving oneself would be no gift.

The contraposition to the Allon is not a theoretically inferred contradiction. Just as we fortify ourselves in getting up over against the world before we seek to command the world practically or theoretically, so too the world is experienced as counter-manding. Just as, in getting up, we set ourselves vis-a-vis the Allon yet remain a part of it, and just as we are able to hear our own voice resounding in the Allon, so that which is our own is not removed from the Allon. The boundaries of the Allon are doubly displaceable: towards the Allon and towards us. In somatic pain we feel the pressure of the Allon overpowering us. In sickness our own body is alienated from us; we realize a foreign power at work within it and try to discover what is going on there within us that makes us suffer. We refer to the fever as *seizing* the patient, to the vertigo as *attacking* him, to the injury as causing him to *succumb*—in brief, we speak of illnesses as if they were entities, alien beings able to possess the sick person. So too do we experience the power of the Allon in the instincts that drive us, as in need and desire, toward gratification.

The boundaries of the Allon are displaceable between the poles of intimacy and strangeness, of belonging and distance, of grasping and being grasped, of mastering and being overpowered. Such shifts of boundaries are experienced, in the extreme pathological case, as derealization or depersonalization, as inspiration or alien influence. The I-Allon relation is always changed as a whole, the particulars fitting themselves into these fundamental changes. The depersonalized patient hears the voice he produces, but no longer hears it as his own. In contrast to the anosognostic he still *knows* that it is his, but the Allon has been shifted into virtually absolute opposition.

At this point clinical psychiatry enters the scene and demands further consideration of its experience with patients, in whom it has established ego-disturbances, ecstasies and depersonalization, thoughts imposed and withdrawn, catatonic movements and automatic obedience. This unforeseen intruding of clinical empiricism into the phenomenological analysis is noteworthy because even though our presentation is guided by the idea that the question of the norm is the basic problem of psychiatry, we began our consideration without any glance in the direction of the clinic. But just as we were previously able to point to anosognosia as an example, so schizophrenic symptoms force their entrance here and call for an initial consideration. Thereby many manifestations stamped irreducible stand to lose that label. It is of course scientifically very unsatisfactory that typical modes of behavior and experiencing, recurring in many cases, should be irreducible.

True, these patients are not accessible to empathy in daily life, and thus they appear "crazy"; yet just such slang expressions implicitly refer to the norms of everyday behavior. The morbid process, the break in the life history, cannot relieve us from the theoretical task of comprehending pathological manifestations as destructions of the norm. Each structure allows only a limited number of possible de-structions. A steel arch cannot be destroyed by fire in the same way as a wooden shed or a tent. Obviously our analysis serves psychiatric practice in revealing the structure of the norm. Since we do not consider the straight path of clinical induction to be the shortest route to an understanding of the abnormal, and since we have thus decided on a lengthy detour, the unexpected vista of the clinic encourages us to follow our chosen path patiently.

In rising up man establishes himself in opposition to the Allon. His position is mundocentric. One might illustrate this by referring to the situation of a person shipwrecked and drifting alone on a raft in the ocean, were it not that such a comparison would evoke the idea of a loss of an original security. The difficulty in finding an appropriate figure stems from the fact that we are trying to describe a basic situation that persists despite all epistructures—not a beginning, once actual but eventually left behind. The situation of the individual is mundocentric insofar as each person experiences the world from his position alone, his "here" being forever surrounded by many "theres". When the former center is left behind, a new one forms immediately. To refer to this basic position the expression "mundocentric" has been coined in analogy, but also in contrast, with "egocentric" and "geocentric". We usually characterize as "egocentric" a person who places himself in the center and deems that everything revolves around him, similar to geocentrical astronomy, which placed the earth in the middle and had the stars revolving around it. Mundocentric, on the other hand, implies that in relation to the world we discover ourselves continually at *a*, but never at *the*, center.

In our mundocentric position we comport ourselves in relation to the Allon as parts to the whole. The familiar conjunction of "parts" and "whole" usually refers to an intelligibly articulated unity, like, say, an organism with its organs or a sentence with its words. As a rule we don't stop to wonder that we are able to grasp the meaning of a whole sentence from the sequence of particular words, or that a physician examines the heart as part of the entire organism. It does not surprise us because it is evident that in such cases a part and a finite whole are seen together by an observer. In our relation to the Allon, however, each one of us, though a part, grasps, in a certain manner, precisely that whole whose order includes him as a part. Applied to the earlier grammatical example this would mean that the particular word is able to comprehend all the other words and the meaning of the entire sentence, an obviously absurd assumption. And yet we speak meaningfully of "the world", "the whole world", "the universe"; more modestly we speak of "the earth", which we state to be round and rotating on its axis, taking us along with it. In saying this, we mean, ultimately, a whole, the terrestrial sphere, of which we form a part—a speck of dust, as it is said. The same relation of a part grasping the whole to which it belongs exists also in ordinary everyday situations that do not require hypothetical explanation. A passenger on a ship or the inhabitant of a house—both in our everyday view of things—have a relationship to the ship as a whole or to the house as a whole. In practice it doesn't seem at all surprising that as parts we are able to grasp, in a particular fashion, the whole to which we belong; upon reflection, however, the relation seems paradoxical and, from a physiological viewpoint, absurd.

The metaphysical speculation of past centuries sought a solution of this problem in the concepts of the microcosm or of the monad, in which the entire universe was said to be mirrored. But the sought-for harmony of opposites, the identification of parts with the whole, is inadequate to express the mundane situation. A mirror mirrors everything save itself; it mirrors for an onlooker, but not for itself. If, like LEIBNIZ, one views the monads as microcosms, each representing the whole universe in different degrees of distinctness, then it is precisely the real relation of man to the Allon, the belonging as a part to a whole and yet the being in contraposition, which is omitted. The search for the harmony of opposites aims "basically" at suspending the tension experienced within the real relation of part and whole. Despite all efforts to master the whole through the mediation of discursive thought or entrusting oneself in faith to the whole, the tension of op-position persists. The Tower of Babel has remained unfinished.

In our relationship to the Allon the whole reveals itself only in fragments. The fragments, comprehended as such, refer beyond themselves to still other fragments and to the constantly present background of the as yet indeterminate whole. We always find ourselves encircled by a spatial and a temporal horizon, which, however open, remains a boundary that excludes what lies beyond it. To the eye aimed at the Allon as a whole things appear as objects (Gegen-stände), their colors as surface colors confining vision [1]. Held by "heft" in the "here" we exchange one particular for another [2]. Within the horizon a focal organization articulates what is distant and what is within reach, so that finally a particular object may be sought, avoided, or neutralized.

---

[1] An allusion to the "surface colors" studied by the Gestalt psychologist, DAVID KATZ. See his: "The world of color". London: Kegan Paul 1935. E. E.

[2] We refer to the phenomena described in psychology under the rubrics of "coarctation of consciousness" and "attention".

Consequently the usual schema of the reflex is, in a way, reversed in the primary situation; for in the schema of the reflex the sensory stimulation precedes the efferent impulse and muscle contraction. Yet this temporal order: first stimulus, then reaction, makes it theoretically impossible that an action—if it were identical with muscle contractions—could ever be directed at an object—if it were identical with stimuli. The reflex is, and remains, an event *within* the organism. In the primary situation, on the contrary, we consider the relation of the living creature to the world. Here the rising up from the ground, the coping with gravity, and the acquistion of freedom of movement take natural priority. Rising from the ground makes object-directed sensory experience possible in the activity of comportment [1]. Distance, detachment, and direction are opened only to creatures essentially motile and no longer bound to a single spot. Sensory experience which, descending from the whole, makes articulation of the Allon and thereby communication feasible, is intrinsically inseparable from motility. This statement is not contradicted by the Bell-Magendie law, as far as that law holds. For a centripetal impulse functions as sensory "input" and a centrifugal impulse as motor "output" only within the integrated organism, which as such must be regarded in its relation to the world.

The proposition that only motile beings are capable of consciousness does not imply however that the "egoic *(ichliche)* motility" (HUSSERL) precedes sensory experience in time. Nor is motility a condition of sensory experience so that, after its work has been done, it may vanish from the scene. Rather, sensory experience remains conditioned throughout by motility, i. e., by actual comportment toward the Allon.

Our primary relation to the Allon is never that of being at a neutral distance. An affective tension is constantly present, a basic tonus that can be neutralized only from time to time and by mediate steps. In getting up man opposes himself as a single individual to the whole; this is reason enough for phobic giddiness to befall him when in a confrontation with openness, depths, abyss, the human situation is revealed. In contrast the narrow twisting passageways of a medieval town, which confine sight, are "gemütlich"; the merciless glare of searchlights is "ungemütlich". "Gemütlich" is the lamp that illuminates a chamber, veiling the surroundings in gentle darkness; outside the room the uncanny lies in wait.

Our analysis of sensory experience, as it forms within the primary situation, does not overstep the limits of the life world, which, to be sure, is also the neglected, silenced, often even contested playground of the natural scientist who claims objectivity. In scientific practice the investi-

---

[1] This concept of the intentionality of sensory experience is not identical with HUSSERL's doctrine of intentionality. To discuss the agreement and the differences would require more space than is available here.

gator, in all his activities of observing, experimenting, and communicating, proves to be a respectable citizen of the life world. There it is taken for granted that he is concerned with objects that exist independently of himself. To such objects, as well as to his scales and instruments, the observer must turn. There is thus a moment of activity inherent in sensory experiencing that is not fully accounted for by the concept of attention.

The psychologist who compares "light stimuli and their neurophysiological or psychophysiological effects quantitatively" never thinks of applying the principles of his method to himself. If he did so, then the visible objects of his observation would be transformed into events that belong simply and solely to the visual system of the observer himself, accompanied somehow—but how remains mysterious—by sensory data. Yet no psychophysics could transform such images back into perceptions of real objects. All "esse" would have been absorbed by "percipi". Even the observer himself would be unable to resist this suction; he would disappear as a bodily subject, along with his entire surroundings, into a solipsistic subjectivity. Paradoxically the requirement of objectivity, the apprehension of objects as such, can be fulfilled only in the life world, and cannot even be meaningfully raised in the reduced world of natural science. Eye and retina, optic nerve and calcarina, ganglion cells and microglia have no relation to objects qua objects; thus they can be neither objective nor subjective. Similarly, no kind of relationship to an object as object can be ascribed to the accompanying sensory data or perceptual images—if there are such images.

Traditionally, sensory experience has been interpreted as purely receptive. The organs of seeing and hearing have been reduced in theory to mere receptors. No one can dispute the right of sense physiology to investigate the eye and ear as instruments. The subsequent step, however, has turned out to be fateful: the attempt to derive the total content of sensory experience from the structure and function of the sensory apparatus and to liken the relation of the one who sees and what can be seen to the reaction of the optical system to photic stimuli. The whole content of sensory experience necessarily suffers a violent mutilation. Since the psychophysics of visual perception has been pre-established by physics in terms of the relation of sender and receiver, the "subjective" data must be accommodated to the objective data. The effect of the sender upon the receptor can be, even at best, only such that the distribution of excitations in the sense organ corresponds to the arrangement of the "stimulus array", just as on a photographic film. The local intensities of photochemical reaction correspond to the distribution of optical energies reflected from the sender. The physiological effect can then be taken as a copy of the acting stimuli. In this sense occasional reference is made quite naively to "retinal images", to which it is assumed the images of perception can be related. Sensory experience is

4*

reduced to the appearance of images in consciousness. Apart from the fact that images are images only for a viewer, and that in unreduced experience we are aware of objects themselves and not of their images, perception is not restricted to the awareness of the objects; we are aware of objects in relation to ourselves in our corporeal existence. Certainly an eye, a retina, or a visual system, is unable to direct itself at anything. Only when the nervous system or consciousness is posited as the effective subject, replacing man or animal in the primary situation, and then only after the theoretical elimination of motility, can sensory awareness be reduced to sheer receptivity. The motile organism, however, does not operate as a mere receiver of stimuli. A creature rising up from the ground is already actively directed towards the Allon. Sensory experiencing is an active attainment and acquisition.

Dilthey's thesis that "our belief in the reality of the external world" derives from the experience of resistance—i. e., resistance to an active expansive motion—may be reversed so that we motile beings experience the Allon, of which we are a part, as resisting [1]. Since we are directed towards the Allon as motile beings we ap-prehend it in hearing and grasp it in feeling and in throwing a glance at things;—the Allon, responding or thwarting our intentions, answers or keeps silent. Colors, tones, scents, all the sensory qualities are not a collection of neutral data; they invariably have a physiognomic character. Metaphors like gay colors, gloomy silence, and sweet music, are to be taken literally. Our contacts with the powerful Allon vary with every sense modality. In the total relation with the Allon certain areas correspond to our intentions while others fail to do so; between the two there are fields of neutrality [2]. The primary distinction is between what is bound by gravity and what is detached, or, in other words, between the perdurable ground and everything motile and autokinetic.

The preceding discussion of the primary situation has given priority to the relation with the Allon over the relation with the heteros. This order is inherently necessary. For you and I do not face each other directly as ego and alter ego. We meet one another in the—common—world. Only because we comport ourselves toward the Allon and because each of us, as a part, has risen up from a common ground, can we enter into communication with one another. In analogy with the Allon we term our partner the heteros, to show, merely by a linguistic relation, that the other fellow, whom we understand, im-parts himself to us as a part of the Allon.

The heteros frees himself as a part from the totality of the Allon, a part which when we call and answer, or are attracted and follow or

---

[1] Cf. HEIDEGGER, M.: Being and Time, p. 249 ff.

[2] Cf. STRAUS, E.: The primary world of the senses. New York: Macmillan 1963.

approach and flee, responds to our action. The relation to the heteros constitutes itself in a meaningful interplay; the basic form of communication is a synkinetic relationship in the polarity of acceptance—as in smiling—or of rejection—as in lips grimly shut. The understanding of expression also precedes the understanding of speech. The mother sings a lullaby to her baby long before it can understand the meaning of words. Animal existence, both in expression and impression, remains limited to pre-linguistic communication.

Synkinesis functions most effectively between members of the same species but is not limited to this condition. Its sphere also extends to the relationships of man to animal and animal to man, and to the community of animals among themselves and their relation to members of the same and different species. Husserl's doctrine of "appresentation" would be applicable, if it is at all, only to the relation of adult humans. How can one expect a baby smiling at her mother, a dog following his master, a hen calling her chicks, to constitute an alter ego in the "primordial sphere" of a stream of consciousness that is peculiar to the infant, dog, or hen? The transcendental ego itself does not belong to the world whose validity of Being it constitutes. It is an "ego absconditus". The encounter with the other fellow, however, does not occur via transcendence into an ego-alien world. We meet one another in the one world common to us both. Whether the relationships are friendly or hostile is not important in this connection. Yet a merely static demarcation is obviously insufficient: a part somehow singled out in the Allon manifests itself as heteros, as partner, only if he comports himself toward, i. e. against, the Allon as a mobile creature, and is able thus to do so toward me or you. Motility does not function as an "external" expression of inwardness but as physiognomic evidence of comportment toward the world. Experience shows the extent to which movement, manifesting activity, guides the identification or misidentification of species and mates, of friend and foe, throughout the animal world. If scarecrows actually scare the birds away, then surely it is through their action as "mobiles" rather than through their half-human form. "Inanimate nature" was discovered late in the history of mankind—witness the child's world of fairy tales and the adult world of myths dominated by gods and demons. Since the primary form of communication is that of synkinesis, only the failure to secure an answer in the mutual interplay of seeking and finding, of attracting and following, provides, within individual experience, the basis for the discovery of inanimate things. All movement is interpreted for a long time as the activity of a living entity. The discrimination of the mobile from the static, of active comportment from mechanical motion, is not accomplished all at once.

During the first few months of the individual's life, the Allon and the heteros are not clearly separated for the suckling, who of course is also a babe in arms. We may assume that the Allon, at the time of nursing, is still wholly embodied in the nursing mother, and experienced pervasively as responsive. Only with the gradual development of motility is the ambit within which responses fail to occur discovered "step by step". The discrimination proceeds parallel with the stages of getting up, in the degree that the child, raising his head, crawling, standing, and walking, secures his own stand, which in normal development one day expresses itself through the pronoun "I". In this early phase, the "my" has the meaning of belonging-to; "my people" do not so much belong to me as I to them. The position within the group conceals the mundocentric position without ever suspending it completely. The extent of the Allon and the mundocentric position are still veiled, but they are often experienced abruptly in the fear of darkness and of being abandoned.

In relations to other persons, in meeting the heteros, a part-to-part relationship originates, within whose mutuality of taking hold and being-held, of questioning and answering, the Allon, in its totality, moves into the background. In such limit-settings a private region is demarcated in the Allon, a home that hides the mundocentric position, until it once again becomes evident in great natural or political catastrophes or with the irruption of psychosis. Even in the most intimate pairing of the "dual mode" the partners remain apart. Each one can enter into an I-thou relationship with many others. Throughout all the variations of the I-thou relationships, however, I remain solus in my relation to the Allon. In the collapse of I-thou relationships we become once more painfully aware of our primary situation.

VI. Disturbances of the Primary Situation

1. Being Awake

Our relation to the Allon and to the heteros makes it comprehensible that every definite disturbance in this relation, every derangement of our standpoint within the whole, threatens the synkinetic community of part with part. To talk together with understanding we must speak the same language. To understand each other in primary orientation the same rules of the game must implicitly apply to all the participants, i. e., the "circum-ambient" order must be grasped by all participants as one and the same, independent of its changing appearance. However much the surroundings of a dog and his master may differ, the dog could not follow his master if streets and intersections, moving and waiting, did not mean the same for both within the bounds defined by the threatening traffic. But how is it possible that the relation to the Allon can be disturbed? How can one's standpoint be "de-ranged"? Is there anywhere in the "life world" an indication of such possibilities of disturbance? We answer this question with an unqualified "yes", for all of us are well acquainted with transformations of our relation to the Allon in our own everyday experience.

The relation to the Allon, as we have thus far considered it, holds only for one who is awake; he alone, in rising up, can detach himself from the ground and, as a motile being, enter into contraposition to the world, finding in the primary orientation his place within it. In the world opened up to him in awakening he can enter into communication with others, man and animal, if they are also awake. One who is awake can guard a sleeper or assault him: the sleeper is at the mercy of the one awake. Life history actually proceeds only upon awakening. Only the waking hours and days enter into the continuity of a meaningfully developing context. And lastly, only those who are awake can manifest psychic disturbances. Therefore sleep therapy, ever since Aesculapius, has been the psychiatric therapy of choice. This is not to say that a sleeping schizophrenic ceases to be ill. Yet, although pulse, respiration, temperature, and somatic measures in general can still be taken from the sleeper, even from the comatose, psychoses go to sleep with the patient. Psychiatry is that part of medicine in which only the waking person manifests morbid conditions. Somatic medicine, of course, also requires the cooperation of the waking patient for the testing of motor, sensory, and other functions. But in such cases being awake is only a necessary condition for testing performance; it is not the focus of the examination, which is always aimed at particular events *within* the organism. In a sleeping paralytic we can occasionally ascertain the presence of a pathological big-toe reflex. But only when he is awake can he reveal his megalomanic ideas. Sleep, punctuating life history, suspends, along with having-the-world or being-in-the-world, both intersubjectivity and psychiatric or neurotic manifestations.

These four aspects of being awake: the primary orientation in the relationship to the Allon, the possibility of communication, the continuity of life history, and the orderliness or disturbance of comportment, are intrinsically related. Only in being awake are we able to separate I and world, mine and not-mine, real present and future possibility, dream and reality.

Waking sensory experience is not merely one among many kinds of "object consciousness" (Gegenstands-Bewußtsein); it is the primary, basic mode of experiencing. Just as remembrance can be realized only in the present, so images as such can be apprehended only in the present as representing something not actually present. The assertion that "objects exist for us either in the form of perceptions or of ideas" [1] is incorrect. For ideas are never present "for us", while perceived objects present to me can

---

[1] JASPERS, KARL: General Pathology. Chicago: Univ. Chicago Press 1963, p. 60.

also be present to others, i. e., to *us,* in our bodily existence. The thing perceived is not just an intentional datum of consciousness but something bodily contraposed: an "ob-ject". That sensory acquaintance is *fundamental* does not imply that it is the *ultimate* in man's I-Allon relations. But neither praise nor dispraise can rob it of its birthright. Even in challenging the testimony of sensory experience we can never abandon it.

Only when we are awake do we sustain a relation to the Allon. To go to sleep we lie down, we give up our stand in the world opposite to it. Yielding to weightiness we sink into deep sleep, renouncing, along with motility, the vigilance of the senses. To be sure, vigilance is not renounced for all senses in the same way: the ears and hearing do not shut themselves off to invading noises as the eyelids and upturned eyeballs exclude the light. An alarm-clock will awaken a sleeper—sometimes easily, sometimes with only great difficulty, depending on the "depth" of his sleep. Contrasting with the often cited example of a mother whose sleep is not interrupted by loud noises coming from the street, but who is awakened by a faint moaning of her baby, are the cases of those overcome by gas, smoke, and fire while sleeping or those who fall asleep at the wheel of their car and drive to destruction without awakening. To be sure, the relationships with the Allon are not broken off but only interrupted in sleep; still most persons trust the alarm clock rather than rely on the "human clock". Even the mother who has been aroused by a slight sound coming from the nursery must first wake up before she can make contact with her child. In awakening we resume our position within the Allon, in opposition to it. All dreams probably belong to the stage of awakening. With the matutinal summons "Time to get up!" rising and awakeness are meaningfully joined together.

It is inadequate to characterize the contrast of waking and sleeping as an antithesis of degree between lucid and clouded consciousness. Although in a certain sense it is justifiable to view clarity of consciousness and loss of consciousness as extremes on a scale of degrees of "clarity", the contrast between these two conditions, i. e., to be awake and to be asleep, is much more radical; for it is not consciousness that wakes and sleeps; in waking and in sleeping both man and animal enter into different relationships to the world and to themselves. The transition from sleep to being awake is a radical change; being awake calls for optimal neural correlations. Thus awakeness, considered as a stance that opposes the world within the world, is not altogether intelligible as a function of a particular "apparatus in the brain", say, the reticular activating system. Awakeness is not a specific function, like seeing, hearing, or walking. Only someone who is awake can see, hear, or walk. Awakeness, however dependent on events within an organism, must not be identified with them.

The possibility of distinguishing being awake and dreaming holds only for the one who is awake. Upon awakening we notice that we have been asleep; while "falling" asleep we never sense that we have been awake. He who is awake knows about his dreaming; but the dreamer does not know anything about his being asleep, nor about his dreaming. To have dreamt thousands of times does not immunize anyone against a recurrence of dreaming. The dreamer is a captive of his dream world. Not before awakening do I realize that a dream has been my dream—"nothing but a dream". The possibility of differentiating the two worlds occurs only in being awake. Awakening, I note that I have been dreaming; our knowledge of a dream is a knowledge of the past, of sleep which has interrupted the continuity of our life history. The dreamer is trapped in the presence of his dream; nor do such scenes form a coherent texture whatever their supposed latent meaning, which becomes accessible only in a waking interpretation. These latent dream thoughts are not less hidden from the dreamer than his own state of dreaming. Awakening, we take up the thread of our historical existence. The dreams of one night, on the contrary, do not continue the dreams of earlier nights in the way that the hours of our waking life join with those past and those to come. We cannot plan our dreams nor "forecast" them. The dreamer neither knows nor disposes of possibilities other than those immediately present. He is unable to draw a clear line between himself and the Allon, having abandoned—by lying down and falling asleep—his stand in opposition to the Allon. Only while awake can one succeed in deciphering the I-world relation [1].

Heraclitus' frequently quoted aphorism that "the waking have one world in common while the sleepers turn each one to his private world" (Frag. 89) is more than a mere description of fact; it points to an essential relation. Only the waking are able to share the world; only in a common world can we meet the other. In antiquity one's own world, the *idios kosmos,* was considered a private, and that meant a deficient, world. Awakeness was deemed superior to sleep and dreaming. It was not so much communication that called for an explanation as its suspension. In the modern concept of the world as external, constituted in and by the subject's "mind", the problem is reversed. Communication thereby becomes a wellnigh insoluble riddle. It seems to me that our account of comportment towards the Allon and the heteros, in their mundane orientation, coincides in many respects with the ancient view.

The antitheses of waking and sleeping, of primary orientation and dreaming, of common and private worlds, may serve us as a paradigm of the possibility of fundamental changes in relation to the Allon as they are actualized in psychosis. But not all our patients are somnambulists. They are not dreaming; they are awake and yet they are turned away from our

---

[1] Cf. STRAUS, E.: Some remarks about awakeness. In: STRAUS, E.: Phenomenological Psychology. New York: Basic Books 1966.

common world. Although their relation to the Allon resembles in a certain way that of the sleeper and dreamer, it is not the same. To understand the essence of psychotic disturbance we must still enlarge our view of the norm that rules the primary orientation of the waking person. And in so doing we continue the discussion of what has gone before.

2. The Forgotten Protasis of Science

Since awakeness is the unalterable condition for all human activities, it is simply taken for granted and accepted as a situation that is not in need of further exploration, not even when sleep and awakeness are the very topics of physiological research. Of course, a psychologist who records the behavior of men or rats, varying the stimuli and reading the scales, must be awake; yet his own awakeness is not to be determined by measurements. It manifests itself through his relation to the world, in an active comportment that makes observations and measurements possible. The alpha-rhythm of an EEG does not reveal anything by itself, whether it characterizes waking or sleeping conditions. Required is an antecedent standardization, established by inductive correlations with subjects whose status as waking or sleeping persons was evident beforehand. The person who is awake is from the very beginning understood as heteros, i. e., as someone able to comport himself meaningfully towards the Allon. Understanding has as its theme the relation of a waking man or animal to the Allon; it fails in the presence of the sleeper. Events within an organism will be explained by scientific methods; comportment to the world must be understood. Although both explaining and understanding tacitly presuppose the awakeness of the investigator, his own waking comportment to the Allon never becomes thematic. Since this presupposition remains implicit, it is conducive to a specious understanding of the comportment of others and finally of one's own and thereby, in fact, of the primary orientation itself.

In everyday life our interest is turned to the objects perceived without much thought being given to the act of perceiving objects; nor is there any pragmatic reason for it to be otherwise; that is, as long as things move smoothly. What arouses our interest is the behavior of objects, persons, or things; they present the unknown, with which we must deal. But this "natural" attitude leads to paradoxical results if it is carried over unmodified to the investigation of experiencing itself. The empiricist, to be sure, claims to recognize only data gained by, or at least confirmed through, experience; yet empiricism is a theory that—since the days of John Locke —has actually ignored *life world* experience and replaced it with metaphysical and epistemological constructs. Hence experience is not considered as opening a relation for man and animal towards the world but is reduced to "mechanics of images" and—in the physiological extension of sensualism—finally interpreted as vacuous side-effect of events in the afferent nervous system. It is postulated that the optical apparatus, when activated from without, yields as a byproduct some kind of chimerical images. Physiology then has the unrewarding task of correlating such merely subjective data, in precise psychophysical correspondence with processes directly accessible to experimentation and measurement [1]. In BARTLEY's account—quoted here as an example typical of the attitude of most scientists working in this field—not man but the eye is deemed seeing. Seeing is identified with the emergence of visual phenomena, although it is never made clear to whom these phenomena may present themselves, nor how they could reveal their relation to "external events", nor how any observer— scientist or not—could ever establish the coexistence of the two series. Since "visual phenomena" are, and necessarily remain, nescient of their causal relation to occurrences in the "outer world", the "experiential outcomes" must be confined to an "inner world" in strictest solipsistic isolation. Yet these phenomena are supposed to provide the basis for our common-sense experience as well as for the scientific exploration of the "outer world". BARTLEY does not divulge how he actually gained such insight, still less how any creature, confined to the presence of visual phenomena, could ever transcend them into an outer world, which in turn encompasses his own inner world besides that of others. BARTLEY silently claims for himself the privilege of the scientific observer who, being confronted as a human being with objects visible to him, does not hesitate to interpret them as stimuli in relation to others. He speaks a language inherited from a long line of scientific ancestors. In the course of centuries an entangled situation, abounding with contradictions, developed. While in this climate biological research still flourished, the comportment of the scientist himself, underlying all experimenting, was seldom raised to the rank of a problem. A detailed account and critique of this development, dating back to the beginning of modern science, is not feasible within the bounds of this essay. Indispensable, however, is a discussion of a few topics related to the basic activities of the scientific observer, in order to uncover at least some of the hidden pre- suppositions and to improve thereby the insight into the norm that is re- quired for an understanding of the pathological. Let us then consider a technique, apparently remote from any suspicion of subjectivity, to show

---

[1] Cf. for example, BARTLEY, S. HOWARD: Central mechanisms of vision: In: Handbook of physiology. Eds. Field, J., H. W. Magoun, and V. V. Hall. Washington, D. C.: Amer. Physiol. Society 1959, Section I, vol I, chapter 30: "Visual phenomena (are) the experiential outcomes of the action of optic pathway, activated by photic radiation". "The fundamental requirement in relating vision to the various phenomena in the optic pathway is for two sets of events to be initiated by the same external event (stimulus)".

how highly sophisticated observers may conceal from themselves essential characteristics of waking experience.

Our knowledge of the structure and function of the nervous system we owe directly or indirectly to microscopy. Thus every statement about the function of the retina, for example, refers implicitly to its histological elements, such as rods and cones, which are inaccessible to direct observation but are revealed through optical magnification. Yet thorough acquaintance with the construction and manipulation of the microscope by no means guarantees corresponding insight into the observer's own performance and accomplishment.

What do we actually mean when we speak about magnification? What is it that is being magnified? Certainly not the tissues stretched over a microscopic slide. When a house is enlarged, when rooms, floors, and wings are added, the existing structure is altered in its own dimensions, just as in the lengthening of a street or the widening of a bridge. A microscopic preparation, on the other hand, remains unaltered. Magnification is not identical with enlargement. When a house has been remodeled the earlier state is gone; after magnification the microscopic preparation remains just at it was. As soon as the preparation is removed from the microscope stage the magnification disappears, only to reappear with each fresh presentation. Thus the temporal order and the sequence of conditions have an entirely different meaning in the two instances. In the enlargement of a house, the sequence of what is seen corresponds to the sequence of what has occurred. However, when we observe a preparation though the microscope, moving from a weak magnification to a stronger one and then back again, it does not mean that one magnification is later than the other, nor that any magnification as such precedes or succeeds the natural size. Thus we make a clear distinction between the temporal order of our acts of experiencing and the temporal structure of the temporal objects experienced; we can accomplish this because being awake we are able to distinguish between the objects of experience and our experiencing of the objects. And that implies that we experience the object *and* ourselves in a precisely determinable relation.

Obviously, both terms, enlargement as well as magnification, refer to a comparison. In the case of the enlargement of a house we compare, in the planning, an anticipated later condition with the one present, and following its completion, the now present condition with one past. In both instances we are comparing a later and an earlier phase. In looking through a microscope, certain configurations are seen in one particular magnitude—in that one and in no other. The image that appears is understood as magnification only through an unusual sort of comparison, viz., with something that, although present, is not in itself visible to the human eye, and never will be. In this sense an image distorted in a certain way, namely as enlarged, is compared with the thing itself, or more precisely with its hidden suchness.

Thus the enlargement is a kind of image, which is nonetheless distinguishable from those painted on canvas, printed on paper, or photochemically prepared on film, in that the microscopic image is indissolubly wedded to the original. We are able to see the original—unenlarged—without the image, but we are never able to see the microscopic image without the presence of the original (except in reproductions, i. e., in a reproduction of the image). Indeed the material of the microscopic image is of a very special sort, since the refraction affects the light rays after they have already traversed the preparation. Looking into the microscope we often have the impression that we are actually seeing the tissue and its structure; at the same time we know all too well that the original is different from the way in which it is seen, that it is not as large as it appears. We lift off the suchness or the eidos from the thing—as we do whenever we produce or observe an image—and submit it to an optical manipulation rooted in the insight that the spatial proportions of any thing may be represented on any scale whatsoever. Through the microscope we raise the hidden structures of the tissue into the visual sphere of the human eye, well aware that this relation is artificial. In the optical enlargement we leave the thing itself unchanged, but make use of an image adapted to human vision in order to acquire an insight into how the object is constituted, apart from any direct relation to a human being. Thus we compare the image actually seen with the "real" structure of the object, which is present only in phantasy—in a sound phantasy, to be sure, but still in phantasy.

The enlargement, like every comparison, requires something as mediation. As mediation we make use of a scale that is seen diplopically, as it were. We relate the apparent magnitude to a concomitant unmagnified one in vision or thought, and realize that a form judged to be 3 mm. long with a magnification of 30 is in "reality" only 1/10 mm. long in relation to the same standard. Just as a frame separates a picture on the wall from its surroundings so that different standards obtain on one side of the frame and the other side of the frame, so the microscopic image contrasts with the surroundings in an abrupt shift from one standard to another. When a microscopic slide is projected, the screen is seen in its natural size while at the same time the cells and fibers appearing on the screen are seen in magnification. The relation of figure and ground, interpreted as a stimulus configuration, is inadequate for comprehending the simultaneity of the two orders. Screen and picture belong to two different orders of the object world of objects; yet as sources of "stimuli"—whether reflected from the illuminated or from the dark section of the screen—they are not different. Whether light is reflected from the surface of a wall or from the surface of a picture upon it cannot be determined by the visual receptors and the optical system. If the visual phenomena, together with the physiological excitations, were to be correlated with the very same external events, as BARTLEY holds, we would know nothing of images and consequently nothing of optical conducting paths.

The microscopic inspection is preceded by the preparation of the specimen. The histologist is able to use the microscope meaningfully only if he interprets his findings with regard to their technical origination. Every histological statement rests on an historical reconstruction. Returning in thought to the past the scientist realizes that the chromatic structure of tissue elements actually seen through a microscope is the enlarged image of a cross-section on the specimen slide, that this stained section is identical in turn with a previously unstained one, that the section has been separated from a block of paraffin wax in which a portion of, say, an eye was enclosed, that the particular eye had been removed previously from the body of an animal, and that the eyes of the species used in the current experiment are of the same kind as the eye viewed through the microscope. The microscopic preparation is the very last stage of a long series of alterations through which the object has passed. Nevertheless, what the microscope presents is understood precisely as the original structure of the tissue. Interpretive viewing of a microscopic image consequently demands a peculiar temporal mobility on the part of the viewer as he moves back and forth in thought between present and past, effect and cause. In the image available at the end of a long and complex process we come to know the histological elements as they belong, uncolored and unenlarged, to the tissue itself. We then relate certain physiological performances or pathological reactions back to these formations. We interpret a tumor, for example, found post mortem, as the cause of abnormal behavior manifested during the patient's lifetime—i. e., the observation of the effect actually precedes the discovery of the cause, as in every "post mortem" examination and also in many, if not all, experimental studies.

Microscopy, the lifting of invisible structures from hidden depths into the realm of visibility, seems to fulfill a basic postulate of logical positivism; yet to be meaningful the microscopic images require a copious commentary provided only by introspection.

3. Intentionality and Causality

With the invention and use of the microscope man crossed the boundaries of primary orientation. The history of glassmaking, of the grinding of lenses, of the construction of telescopes and microscopes, extends over many hundreds of years. Nevertheless, the capacity to see things as magnified is rooted entirely in the primary orientation. One can therefore demonstrate the phenomenon of magnification to a child in its early years.

Without any specific instruction he (or she) will spontaneously recognize as magnified an object seen through a magnifier. He will be amazed by the details made visible to him without wondering at his own achievement. We all need to learn walking and talking; but the seeing of a magnification does not need to be learned and does not even impress a person as his own achievement but appears rather as awareness of the visible itself. If one has a child observe some object, for example an ant, first with the naked eye and then placed under a magnifying glass, the child will immediately relate the one view to the other. It will recognize in the magnified image the same object that it has previously seen in its natural size. In playing with the magnifying glass, the stimulus patterns, AB, AB, and the views, CD, CD, follow one another in time, yet the child, like all of us who understand a magnification as magnification, sees one and the same thing in the passage of the appearances, now this way, now that, now enlarged, now in natural size.

The discrepancy between the naive accomplishment and the theoretical account indicates that the perception of magnification is merely a variation of the waking orientation to objects in general. Hence, as simple as it appears to demonstrate the phenomenon of enlargement to a child, it nevertheless remains difficult for us as adults to "re-cognize" what has taken place in such a naive performance, the more so since we are inclined to continue the *life-world approach* toward objects. Even so, the self-forgetfulness of investigators devoted to objective methods is often surprising. Every statement about the behavior of things necessarily contains an implicit reference to the behavior of the observer, no matter whether we are dealing with scientific experiments or everyday occurrences. Sensory physiology, psychophysics and behavior research cannot claim a privileged status, or can do so only insofar as it is erroneously postulated that in the long run experimental studies of organisms will provide a complete understanding of perceiving itself. In other words, the relation of the seeing eye—or rather person—to visible objects, is erroneously identified with the relation of an eye as it is seen to photic stimuli. Behavior research, old and new, shudders at merely subjective data; it postulates that human and animal behavior must be explicable as manifestation of events within an organism as—schematically expressed—motor reactions to sensory stimuli. If this doctrine were generally valid, then it would also be applicable to the observer himself. Yet at the very moment such an attempt is made, the house of cards collapses; for then the observer's statement turns out to be nothing but his own verbalizations, his motor response to optical and acoustic stimuli which, emitted from the experimental subject, have excited his receptors. What he claims to have observed objectively in others are, to follow his own line of interpretation, "nothing but" introspective sensory data, caused by photic stimulation. The event observed has been absorbed into the neural processes of the observer and has thereby lost the character of objective observation and of a survey of objects.

Boring and other adherents of operationalism have held that one could at least exclude any consideration of the subjective experience of the experimental subject. The method that ascertains a "discriminatory response" is supposed to free us from idle preoccupation with the subject's experiences. In the term "discriminatory response", however, discriminating acts and discriminated reactions are commingled. The actual operation of discrimination is in fact carried out by the observer, who correlates and compares temporally separated "stimuli" and "responses", in order to discriminate them. It is really an introspective achievement of the observer to unite the suchness of events that are and remain actually separate in their objective existences. The subjective experiences that were to have been eliminated by objective methods inexorably return as modes of the observer's conduct, no matter what the particular object of his observation.

Thus the question once more arises: how can the observer reach the object of his observation? In examining the "light reflex", the examiner, who has determined the pupillary reaction of a patient, enters the usual notation in the patient's record. No reference is made to the observer, although he too must have been affected by the events observed and his own receptors aroused. The examiner does not relate the light reflex of the patient to that bundle of light rays which have impinged on him, the observer. That would be truly absurd; the optical stimuli that caused the pupils of the patient to contract never did reach the observer's rods and cones. But his own pupillary reactions go just as unnoticed. Certainly the patient's reactions that are noticed by an observer are not those of the observer himself. Yet the patient's pupillary reaction could not be tested if light reflected from the surface of the patient's eye had not reached and stimulated the retina of the observer. The statement that a stimulus X has, in an organism O, triggered a reaction Y is based on the comportment of the examiner, who for his part, has reacted to the total situation $X \rightarrow O \rightarrow Y$.

If in the observed process X was a stimulus for O, decided first by the response Y, then the whole configuration and sequence $X \rightarrow O \rightarrow Y$ must have been one stimulus-configuration for the observer.

The responses of the observed organism are first defined by and formulated through the responses of the observer. The observed behavior is encompassed by that of the observer. When an observer of an experimental subject distinguishes "in-put" from "out-put", then, in relation to himself, the whole articulated event is—viewed physiologically—"in-put". The two series do not run parallel. When light, reflected from the subject's body during the two phases of in-put and out-put, has been absorbed by the observer's receptors, what else could it, according to the theory, instigate, except motor responses in the observer's body? In the stimulated organism efferent impulses follow the afferent ones in time; they do not refer back to the releasing stimuli, let alone to the stimuli sources. Still, the experimenter speaks only of objects; his findings, and protocol statements, deal with the Other; they deal on a macroscopic level with men and rats, with animals and things, and their relationship to one another. The observer relates the "response" of the subject back to the "stimulus" that preceded it, contrary to the direction of the objective passage of time. Only through such a "re-course" can an event be grasped as a "re-sponse", a "re-action" to a preceding event, and only through such a re-course can the preceding occurrence be comprehended as releasing.

In every observation of human and animal behavior two organisms, two nervous systems, are engaged. What is sauce for the goose ought to be sauce for the gander. Yet in the physiology of the senses, in the study of behavior, two different standards are usually applied. The experience of the subject is referred to a physically reduced surrounding by an observer who does not and cannot surrender his standpoint in the everyday-life world. The observer sets himself above the law that is supposed to be universally binding. Causal and intentional relationships are radically separated and in perfect discretion distributed between the subject observed and the observer himself. The subject's behavior is interpreted as responses to stimuli and recorded by an observer whose own object-intentional attitude remains completely unconsidered, nay, whose own observer-role is simply ignored. Yet the observer himself must be affected by the events that he describes. He must be included in the overall process of the observing. The observer is just as involved in the entire event as the one observed. In his protocol statements to be sure, he disinvolves himself, without any concern for his ineluctable involvement or for the possibility of and justification for such disinvolvement. Psychiatry furnishes striking examples of the extent to which disinvolvement can fail. We have no reason in such cases to register the experience of being affected as something entirely novel and incomprehensible, although there is cause to ask why the normally tacit functioning of such disinvolvement breaks down.

In observing, as in sensory experience generally, we stand in a twofold relation to things. We are affected by them, and in being affected by them, we grasp them as objects. The question is how the causal relation ties in with the intentional relation, whether the latter can and must be reduced to the former, whether, therefore, the one can be interpreted as real, the other as merely apparent, or whether and in what manner an integration is thinkable. It is not enough to refer, with KANT, to an "affection of the sensorium" or with HUSSERL to "hyletic" material animated by meaning-constituting acts. Nor is it at all sufficient to grant, willy-nilly, an intentional consciousness to one's fellow man and to forget that we, the observers, directed to what is objectively given, are ourselves affected by the object of our observation. As an observer, I am, like everyone, affected in my own bodily being by light and sound, i. e., by stimuli. Such being affected is the condition of my perception of objects. Nevertheless, the stimuli impinge on me as a motile creature. This motility is, however, not merely the *conditio sine qua non* of sensory experience; it is not just a condition which must be fulfilled in order for other events to occur, comparable to buying a ticket, that will enable the owner to enter the concert hall and thereby be affected by sound waves. In rising against gravity the fundamental relation to the Allon is coarctated and therewith is first established the distance to be bridged afterwards by sensory experience. Without that distance contact would not be possible. As motile beings we see and hear by means of the eyes and the ears. Sensory experience is not the summation and end result of the functions of sensory instruments; it is not made up of particular stimulus-bound world-less data; it is not mere "reception". In rising against gravity we launch ourselves into a situation of being affected. Awake, we potentially present ourselves to a forthcoming stimulation. The circumstances will determine the details we must experience here and now, whenever we open our eyes, direct our gaze, and face the environment. Sensory experience is neither completely receptive nor completely active. The stimulus actualizes and thereby determines and confines, in its suchness, what is potentially accessible in the total I-Allon relation. While stimuli materially impinge on the "receptors", objects as such appear to us. The Colosseum, the Eiffel Tower, stand in their places, visible to all of us together. The buildings are not physically absorbed by the spectators; the light reflected from their surfaces, however, diverges in many bundles of rays, of which only a few, passing through the narrow opening of a pupil, will become effective as stimuli. A thousand viewers receive a thousand stimuli, just as a thousand hungry mouths require a thousand portions of food to be satisfied. Stimuli, like servings of food, are incorporated. Yet while nobody is able to share stimuli with other people, we have the sight of visible objects in common. Food, once consumed, cannot satisfy us a second time, but we can see the objects once again in their suchness as the other.

In the glare of light, we experience the necessity to perceive and the power of the perceived. When light fades, when every sound is stilled, still the Allon confronts us, in darkness and silence, gloomy and brooding. In the primary orientation we experience the Allon as "counter-part"; invariably it has a physiognomy.

In the relation of the one seeing to the visible, outer world and inner world are not separated. Consequently, no effort is required to join the divided realms. No dichotomy of body and soul is to be healed here. The relation of the see-r to the visible cannot be reduced to the relationship of stimuli and receptors.

4. The Bipolarity of Experiencing

In order to halt the fateful confusion of stimulus and object, we would like to demonstrate their disparity, using as an example an activity familiar to all of us from everyday life—the card game. Let us compare the relation of a player to his cards, considered as objects, with the relationship of his receptors to stimuli. The players handle the cards, flat pieces of cardboard that pass from hand to hand. Each card—still considered as an object—has two sides, a front side with an individual "face", which distinguishes each one from all the others, and a reverse side, which shows a design, the same one on all cards. As a rule, each card is named and handled according to its "face value", King of Clubs, Queen of Diamonds, etc., even when, viewed from the back during a game, it is not recognizable as such. Front and back are indissolubly wedded in the object, although they are never visible simultaneously. *Experientially* the one side invariably disappears from our sight whenever the other one appears. This can be tested as often as one likes; the outcome of this trivial experiment remains unchanged. Front and back sides are never present to us at the same time, and yet we are convinced that they are coterminous. Consequently, our conception of the object as such cannot be derived from the sequence of single impressions.

But in line with the tradition that reaches back to DESCARTES, LOCKE, and HUME, our knowledge of things in the "outer world" supposedly stems from discrete stimulus-bound impressions. A sequence of impressions supposedly corresponds to the sequence of stimuli, and our ideas of the concomitance of events in the outer world supposedly correspond to the juxtaposition of particular impressions. Such a correspondence is not to be detected in dealing with playing cards. Our vision of the thing stands in uncompromising contrast to the sequence of sensory data. The factual discrepancy between the comprehended order of things and the order of comprehending acts is not at all difficult to discover, as the card game shows. There can be no doubt that the players are fully aware of it, for the co-existence of the two sides of a single card—despite the actual concealment of one of the two sides—is the very nerve center of the game; it is the "condition of its possibility".

On the level of direct views, stimuli do not figure as a topic of conversation. Stimuli are invisible; physically defined, light neither shines nor shows "all the colors of the rainbow". That colored wall over there is an object of my vision; it is not a stimulus for my receptors [1]. The photons, reflected

---

[1] SHERRINGTON, in his late work: "Man on his Nature", has given us a masterful treatment of these problems. But his version of human nature is constricted by a radical opposition of energy and mind and by a divorcing of the solipsistic mind, which receives perceptual images, from its object world.

from the wall, are, at the moment when they hit the wall, not yet stimuli; they act as stimuli only after having reached and aroused a receptor. Stimulus and organism do not exist separate from one another. Thus, it would be more correct to speak of stimulations than of stimuli, in order to avoid the radical confusion pervading present conventional usage of the word stimuli, erroneously applied to objects, but considered by the observer as possible sources of stimulation. The observer, never suspending this every-day-life attitude, explores the relationship of one object—the organism—to other objects, only to interpret this relationship thereafter in physical and physiological concepts. In the reduced world of physics, however, receptors have no relations to objects as such[1]. The customary confusion occurs because the reduction is not carried through rigorously. Still, it must be maintained that stimulations and subsequent excitations occur, in each instance, *within* an organism where they succeed one another in objective time. If one considers the physiological events as real ones, underlying and determining experience, then a stricter correspondence between stimulus and impression is called for, but then the distinction of the two temporal orders in a card game would be incomprehensible.

When a card is turned from its face to its back a stimulus configuration "B" takes the place of "F". We, of course, are aware of both positions; but "F" knows nothing of "B", which has not yet occurred; likewise "B" knows nothing of a preceding "F". While objects passing through temporal modifications remain the same in the process for us, single stimuli follow each other in rapid succession; if they were recorded on a fast moving film, each one of them would appear on a frame at a definite distance from any other. We integrate F and B in the sequence FB, but the impression of succession cannot be derived from the succession of discrete stimulus effects in time.

If the two sides of a card were photographed on a film strip, then F would produce a photochemical effect on a frame A, and B would produce one on a separate frame, Y. In projecting this film, the spatially distinct frames would also be brought before the lens one after the other. If the order of what is seen corresponded to the order of the stimulations, we would be in no position at all to grasp the sequence of impressions.

But haven't we failed to consider one crucially important factor, namely, the turning over of the card? Isn't it simply this act of turning over that "suggests" to us the idea of the concurrent presence of front and back sides? We notice that, with each turning, F disappears while B appears, and thus we come gradually to the insight that F and B must belong together intimately. The action of turning, however, already implies an object with

---

[1] In fact, it is doubtful whether it is still justified to speak — after the reduction — about organisms, receptors, and brains conceived on a macroscopic level.

front and back sides, an object that remains identical while it is being turned over, and thus able to be "re-turned" by a later turn to its initial position. An advancing in time is in this case a reversion to the beginning.

None of the features that define the cards as objects for the player recur in the relation of stimulus and receptor, or, more properly speaking, can be directly rooted in this relation. If the card is turned over from front to back, then the stimulus configuration B succeeds that of F. The cards are turned, the stimuli are not; stimuli are merely groups of rays reflected from the cards at each moment. All our life long however, the light that arouses the retina enters our eyes from one and the same direction only. Within the visual system and its afferent passageways there is no forwards and backwards; there is a centripetal direction only. Of the object that reflects the light the retina knows nothing. What has happened to the light before it reaches a receptor is irrelevant for it. The stimulus, understood as such, has no history. Stimulation is limited entirely to the actual moment of the local effect. Just as optical stimuli move along a one-way street, as it were, so also the excitation towards the calcarina is conducted exclusively in a single direction. Neither optical stimuli nor excitations are turned over, nor are sensory data. Nor could the hypothetical perceptual images be turned over, for images of that sort, although presumably representing spatial relations, are not themselves figures that occupy terrestrial space. Furthermore, the total scene of table and cards would not be turned over, but only one part in relation to other parts and to ourselves. The turning of a card has no analogue in cerebral events.

Turning a card over is a simple action. We see the object, reach for it, take hold of it, and turn it over with a twist of the wrist and hand. "We stretch out our hand for the card" means that in the present moment we see the object as a possible, i. e., a prospective, goal before us, corresponding to the direction of our glance, but not to the direction of the entering light. The muscle contractions released in an organism by optical stimulation are, however, directed to naught else, to no goal; they succeed the stimulation. The motor effect—if it could reach at all—would reach into a void. We reach out our hand toward a visible object; the motor reaction does not bring the hand into contact with optical stimuli. When *we* touch and grasp a visible object, the thing touched is identical with the one seen; tactile stimulation, however, always follows in the wake of the visual separated by two "syn-apses". The comportment of the players has no one-to-one correspondence with sensori-motor events in the organism.

Card games are social events in which a number of persons participate. While the cards are visible to all of them in common, the stimuli enabling them to play together affect each organism singly. The excitations of one organism do not participate in those of another. The players see the cards in changing positions and identify them as the same when they see them again.

They know that while a card in their own hand shows them its face, it turns its back to their fellow players. While the cards persist throughout the process of shuffling as the self-same individuals, the stimuli are not shuffled, nor do they retain their identity through the passage in time. As physical events, stimulations never return. "Seeing again" necessarily implies temporally separated excitations and temporally separated visual acts. When we see something again the temporal interval and the discreteness of the impressions are not effaced. Indeed the very condition of "re-cognition" and identification is that the first event is already past, and is separated by a shorter or longer interval from the later one. In "seeing again" we are aware that what is seen at present has already shown itself to us previously, then disappeared from sight, and now reappears. Particular stimulations, which follow one another in objective time, are unable to comprehend their temporal interrelations. A stimulation is unable to compare itself with another one as later; the earlier one is unavailable to it. In "seeing again" we actually experience ourselves in relation to the Allon, experiencing within the stimulus-conditioned here and now the relationship of present to past. Carried along on the stream of time from moment to moment, we experience our relationship to the Allon within the horizon of historical time.

The fundamental diversity of stimuli and objects can be demonstrated easily and forcefully if one does not refuse to consider the phenomena in their unabated fullness. Yet it cannot be denied that, despite all discrepancy, there must be a connection. Our everyday-life experience depends on the excitation of our sense organs. To this proposition: "While objects are turned before our eyes, stimuli are not turned," corresponds the correlative: "Although the stimuli are not turned, the visible objects are turned." We cannot stop with merely determining a deficiency; we must still try to comprehend the richness of "life-world" experience. Thus the next question is: How is it possible to account for the fact that our experience so far transcends the processes explorable by physiology?

The answer to this question has of course been anticipated in our entire presentation up to this point. We have tried to remove the strait jacket in which epistemological and scientific traditions have bound the observer of the *life-world*. We have sought to describe the relation of experiencing creatures to the experienced world and to comprehend this relation without prematurely reducing it to physiological processes. Consequently we have not referred to a nervous system that projects sensory data into consciousness like a mirage. Nor do we posit a subject of consciousness reaching enigmatically out into an external world and just as enigmatically being affected by it. We have shown that the relation of creatures to the living world is rooted in the organization of the *lived* body, i. e., in the nature of man and animal. The mundane subject, itself a corporeal part of the world, opposing the Allon as a motile being, distinct while belonging to it, has replaced the traditional extramundane subject of consciousness. Stimuli excite the receptors of an organism already steadily directed towards the Allon. Eye and ear function as sensory organs only insofar as they are integral parts of such a terrestrial creature.

In seeing we are turned towards the world. The direction of our gaze is opposed to the movement of the entering light and to centripetally conducted excitation, a fact which deserves to be taken seriously and which cannot be accounted for by the silly hypothesis of external projection. The direction of gazing is inherent in sensory orientation; it is indispensable for sensory orientation; though the direction of gazing is itself unseen, only with it do objects as such become visible to us. If we restrict ourselves to a consideration of the "world of colors", then it may be legitimate to speak of "surface colors". "Surface" is a colored plane, but, only as *one* face of an object that presents itself to us as a many-sided thing and only insofar as we ourselves face the Allon as motile creatures. The act of seeing contains more than what can be represented in a purely optical analysis. The forward direction of the glance is rooted in the motoric "forward", and that means, in the final analysis, in a relation to the Allon. We experience "beaming" light, to be sure, as in agreement with the physical direction of light, but even then we still experience it as coming from over there, from the light source. It moves towards us from the Allon, just as a glance from over here may "pierce" us [1]. If the intensity of the beaming light is increased, then—without any change in the functioning of the sensory apparatus— epicritic vision reverses into protopathic blindness. In pain, when overpowered by the thrust of the Allon, we are unable to preserve our autonomy, we "lose our senses".

Sensory experience is bipolar. We grasp the structure of the Allon and ourselves in relation to it. How could it be otherwise? How else could we orient ourselves in the world and direct ourselves accordingly in our comportment? In walking, we experience ourselves as moving and the streets and houses as being at rest. We master the visible distance in many disparate steps. Players in the card game are clearly aware, without the least forethought, of a dual temporal order: simultaneity in the object and sequentiality of perceptions. They leave it to us to marvel at such lofty

---

[1] Sensory physiological experiments have recently made plausible the hypothesis that centrifugal excitations also occur in the sensory systems. If these findings should be confirmed, it would not change the basic situation at all. For it still remains unexplained that our glance is opposed to the direction of the entering light. Efferent impulses are not sufficient for such an explanation, for two reasons: 1) The comprehension of direction already implies the anticipation of a goal, and 2) In seeing we are directed toward objects as to the Other. Centrifugal as well as centripetal processes, on the other hand, take place within an organism.

banalities. Evidently the player grasps the thing as seen in relation to himself as the one who sees. He realizes his relation to the Allon as the relationship of a part to the whole, which is only to be explored in discursive steps. That is to say that each moment is a phase in a temporal continuum; each single moment points to other ones, past and future, for its completion.

The four walls of a room in which we feel cozy and protected, our own four walls, are never seen simultaneously as they are represented on a blueprint. Our view is always restricted to one part of the space, the whole is never grasped *in one glance*. Whenever we turn one section disappears, another emerges. Nevertheless, it is clear to us that two such sections belong together, that they coexist. The order of visible space does not correspond with the temporal order of our views, nor these again with the order of stimuli. So, although we never see a room as a whole with our eyes, yet we comport ourselves toward it as a whole. With each turn one part alone becomes visible, but we let the parts fuse together as fore and rear views, according to "what matters". Each section will dovetail without further ado; no particular effort is necessary, no reflection, no inference. Children and animals accomplish this task so effortlessly that it never occurs to anyone it could happen differently.

BERKELEY should have broadened his argument—namely, that spatial distance cannot be grasped by vision—to say that a segment of space cannot be grasped visually as a whole, because the two opposite halves are never seen in contraposed directions. After each 180 degree turn of the glance, what is seen lies before the eyes. The site of the window and the opposite rear wall of a room are projected upon the retina in successive phases, but without a change in direction of the incident light. Nay, the discrepancies between optical data are still more radical, for with each turn of the body the relation of the right and left parts of the surroundings are transposed. In our experience the front half of the right side wall of the room is continuously joined to its rear half, notwithstanding the fact that it appears on the left after a 180 degree turn and furthermore that in the optical projections the right and left visual fields, with their corresponding locations upon the retinae, the cortical pathways and areas have been switched. Despite such drastic modifications of physiological conditions we do not join the one half of one wall to the opposite half in our perception. The continuity of what is seen is preserved with the other constancies of size, color, etc. Accordingly, we have no difficulty in recognizing a street, passed through in the direction A → B, as the same on our way back, although in terms of stimuli and cortical projections right and left, near and far, have been transposed. Thus we realize not only that we walk along the same street with its own order of houses and their juxtaposition unaltered, but also that we are moving in a reversed direction.

In the primary orientation we experience ourselves in a mirror of the Allon and therefore are able to recognize ourselves in a mirror. The axes of a room do not turn with the turning of our gazes. Only in relation to such a system reposing in its "heft", will our own turning be graspable; in this relation of a moving part and a resting whole the frame of reference is not a matter of choice. With an acceleration of rotation—particularly one passively induced and no longer compensated for by vestibular reactions—the threshold is soon reached where the separation of the two orders breaks down, where we become dizzy and are no longer able to hold ourselves upright, while at the same time the order of the surroundings disintegrates before our eyes in a chaos of fragmentary impressions.

5. The Symptomatic Psychoses

Our relation to objects and the relationship of stimuli to receptors are incommensurable. The doctrine espoused by BARTLEY, directly correlating visual phenomena and stimuli, corresponds at best to extreme pathological conditions. A world constructed throughout in terms of stimuli would be a mad world. Actually it is a mad world, or more politely expressed, one of a variety of conditions clinically termed symptomatic psychoses, where, with the breakdown of primary orientation, stimulus-bound events become dominant.

The connection is this: the possibilities given by motility first reach full fruition in awakening. In sleep and awake man and animal are bound to the terrestrial rhythms of night and day. But the transition from sleeping to waking is not, as in the plant realm, a mere shift from one phase of vegetative activity to another. In waking up we first come to ourselves, i. e., achieve a stand and a capacity for action in contraposition to the Allon. In awakening, the shutters to the world are flung wide open. When we are awake we are doers, but the awakening itself is not our deed; we wake up by the grace of the *lived body*. To be awake calls for an optimal coordination of somatic functions. Consequently, many drugs, for example LSD, are able to produce far-reaching changes even in minimal doses, through a disturbance of the pattern of correlations. Only when our "op-position" towards the ground has been firmly established do we gain that distance which allows objects to appear in their own structure and *gestalt;* then, incorporated into this universally valid order, we are first enabled to meet others and to communicate with them as partners.

Symptomatic psychoses are modi of experiencing between the poles of awakeness and coma, denoted in clinical parlance as a "clouding of consciousness", a condition considered by many investigators as their central feature. In our view, the clouding of consciousness is not merely a single, although indispensable, symptom, to which secondary symptoms may be added. With every disturbance of the primary orientation, the I-Allon relation is altered in all its component parts.

The status and significance of the "clouding of consciousness" did not remain uncontested. What *is* disputed is the factual justification for taking it as the cardinal symptom; some observers insist that there are somatic psychoses where a clouding of consciousness cannot be demonstrated. Even more radical is the attack on the concept of the clouding of consciousness itself. CONRAD—too early departed—pointed out in his profound presentation of symptomatic psychoses [1] the predicament of the theorists in trying to define consciousness as such and the embarrassment resulting from the failure of any attempt to define its clouding conceptually. "For no one can really make clear what he actually understands by the consciousness that is said to be clouded." To be sure, to define consciousness in itself, "wandering lonely through the world" like the Morgensternian "knee" [2], would certainly be very difficult. Yet it is by no means as difficult to give a definition of the conscious human being [3]. Hence CONRAD says—perhaps without being completely clear about the presuppositions and consequences of his own statements: "Unconsciousness is a *man* (my italics) who has come to be, so to speak, 'without world'." CONRAD then adds, "As soon as be begins again 'to have world', that which we are accustomed to term consciousness also begins again." The having of the world is, then, coarcted to a field of experiencing. In symptomatic psychoses, CONRAD writes, the field varies "between the one extreme of complete, waking, bright, and clear articulation ... and the other extreme of complete deformation". With this formulation, however, sick persons as well as healthy ones appear as mere spectators of a field of experience.

Obviously, in this context everything depends on how the "having of world" is understood. In Kraepelinian as well as in Freudian psychiatry this interpretation was decisively affected by the Cartesian dichotomy, and still more by his anthropology. For Descartes insisted that in man, and in man only, the two radically different, finite substances are mysteriously joined, a union manifested in the "Passions de l'âme". Broadly understood, the term "passions" refers to all the affections of the soul, especially to sensations, and in a narrower sense only to the emotions. The expression "passions" indicates that, being tied to the body, the soul has suffered a loss of its complete sovereignty; it is drawn into the bodily process and

---

[1] Psychiatrie der Gegenwart, vol. II, p. 369 ff. Berlin-Heidelberg-New-York: Springer 1960.

[2] MORGENSTERN, CHRISTIAN: Collection of poems. Authorized English version by A. E. W. Eizen. Wiesbaden: Insel-Verlag 1953.

[3] Cf. STRAUS, E.: Norm and pathology of I-world relations. Dis. nerv. and mental disease, Mono. Suppl. 22, 1—12 (1961). Also in Phenomenological Psychology. New York: Basic Books 1966.

subjugated to it. And yet the soul is presumed to direct the body in a sovereign manner through the exercise of free will. In the subsequent elaboration of the Cartesian philosophy the doctrine of free will was abandoned; but in the same measure DESCARTES' conception of the "passions of the soul", i. e., of the dependency of psychic activity on sensations, bodily needs and drives (the "id") gained in significance. Consciousness, which DESCARTES was the first to identify with the soul, degenerated, in the empirical sciences, into a shadow of bodily events. While bodies in the physical world affect one another, there can be no contact between their shadows. A psychic life is attributed to the individual organism, but it is an inner life, conceived as radically individuated, confined to itself. Even though the reality of the "outer world" is not seriously doubted, it is considered to be remote from any direct contact, posited only by judgment, or supposed to be "out there" on the basis of other indices, for example, "reality testing". According to this doctrine, the world is not opened to the experiencing being in his conscious experience; on the contrary, the particular creature is taken as a microcosm which is directed, as a psychic subject in his inner life, exclusively toward the contents of his own consciousness.

In antiquity, the private world of sleepers and dreamers, the *idios kosmos,* was considered deficient in contrast to the world common to all of us—the *koinos kosmos.* In the modern view, the opposition between the shared and private worlds has been obscured, if not obliterated [1]; supposedly there are only private worlds, microcosmoi: the experiencing creature does not find himself in the world; the world has become an enclave of consciousness [2]. The clouding of consciousness has consequently been characterized as "a change in the hierarchical order of simultaneous or successive conscious contents" (BUMKE), or as a "transitory interruption of the continuity of psychic events" (MAYER-GROSS) [3].

The concept of the clouding of consciousness acquires an entirely different importance when the clouding is taken as a manifestation of a disturbance of the primary situation. Instead of continuing to torture ourselves in the vain effort to define consciousness, we will define as

---

[1] Cf. CONRAD: "In truth the waking person finds himself in the perceived landscape, just as the dreamer does in the dreamt one." Psychiat. Gegenw. vol. II, p. 378.

[2] HEIDEGGER was the first to challenge the traditional concept of consciousness in his *Being and Time.* He avoids, however, using the term "consciousness" in his writings, because, as he says, the being of consciousness remains ontologically obscure. HEIDEGGER's "being-in-the-world" is to be understood as *existentiale* and therefore restricted to human being (Dasein). HUSSERL repeatedly mentions waking comportment in his treatment of the *life world,* yet he also did not offer a more detailed analysis of being awake.

[3] See JAHRREISS, W.: Störungen des Bewußtseins. (Disturbances of consciousness.). In: Handbuch der Psychiatrie, I. Berlin: Springer 1928.

experiencing an organism that is able, in its own motility as body-subject, to grasp the Allon as the Allon; we will define as conscious a human being who is able to direct himself to the whole of which he is himself a part. No longer is the attention—"sicklied o'er with the pale cast of thought"— confined to a study of the organization of the fields of experience. The primary order, which is disturbed in a clouding of consciousness, is much more than a hierarchy "of simultaneous or successive conscious contents". What is disturbed is the relation of a man to the world in his manifold relationship to the Allon.

The fundamental features of the I-Allon relationship may now be summarized as follows:

1. In rising up against gravity motile beings, man or animal, effectuate the I-Allon relationship. The expression "Allon" indicates the unique character of this relationship: that of being together in contraposition. I belong to the Allon, and yet detach myself from it. *Within* the world we counter the world.

2. Sensory experience is embedded within this relation to the Allon. The Allon is present to me as body-subject; within my active resistance to gravity the Allon is experienced in its own "heft" and substantiality as resistant, even while in contraposition it is grasped in its suchness as object.

3. Through the several sense modalities we are directed toward the Allon, which reveals itself as the same within the manifold of sensory aspects [1].

4. In standing up, *my* here is constituted in contraposition to the many theres, the range of possible future whereabouts.

5. In our "auto-nomy" vis-a-vis the Allon we are never radically separated from it. In breathing and eating we remain in continual exchange with the Allon. We remain a part of it. Just as we see other things so we may see ourselves in part; just as we hear the voices of others, so we hear our own words.

6. The boundaries are displaceable. I reach out into the Allon and am dominated by it in my being as body-subject, in my needs and drives. Reaching out into the Allon, I can claim an area there as my own. In illness and in pain I am attacked and overpowered by the Allon. My own body is mine, and yet it also belongs to the Allon.

7. The relation of a motile creature to the Allon is that of a part to an encompassing whole. In the past men were content to ascertain that man sees and hears—and, besides that, moves; that he thinks and plans—and, besides that, moves; that he enjoys and suffers, fears and hopes—and besides that, moves. The simple evidence of facts should suffice to make

---

[1] Cf. STRAUS, E.: Aesthesiology and its significance for an understanding of hallucinations. In: Existence. Angell, May & Ellenberger (Eds.). New York: Basic Books 1958.

clear that motility cannot be a mere addition to sensation, thinking, and feeling. It is as motile creatures that we sense, think, suffer, and hate. With motility a basic situation is created that thematically determines all perceiving, thinking, and feeling.

In rising up, we experience, in solitary mundocentric position, the Allon in its own might, threatened by it and sheltered within it. Our stand within the Allon is precarious; we must continually assert ourselves to counter it. We are always affected by the Allon in one way or another. The relationship to the Allon is first and foremost never one of assembling neutral sense data. The Allon shows itself in a physiognomic pattern, attracting or repelling in particulars, swaying and awful as a whole. From this primary situation the elementary affects emerge as variations of the I-Allon relationship.

8. Hunger, thirst, and all the necessary daily chores mercifully confine our sight to what lies near at hand.

9. The relationship to the Allon is bipolar. In placing ourselves at a distance from what lies opposite to us, we apprehend a twofold order: the objective order in its suchness and invariances, and at the same time the order of our own comportment toward it.

10. In rising up from the ground, we overcome heft but partially. The objective order thus unfolds only in the sequence of our steps. The order of the Allon shows itself as one, valid and binding for everyone.

11. The relation of the part to the whole enables the "im-parting" of communication. Out of the totality of the Allon the heteros stands forth for me, in synkinetic correspondence to my own comportment. There can only be communication, the Allon can mediate only between the one and the other, insofar and as long as it is grasped by all "parti-cipants" in its own structure.

This richly structured order of the primary orientation in waking existence disintegrates in the symptomatic psychoses. The destruction is, however, no mere quantitative loss of clarity and distinctness; it passes through various phases of transformation, ending in a distortion which can be understood only in relation to the norm. A "clouding of consciousness" now means, among other things, that the keeping of distance and the articulation of the polar order fails, that the boundaries toward the Allon are shifted, and that the objective order begins to totter. If and when distantiation fails, then we are delivered up to the Allon, experiencing its power physiognomically as a growing menace.

Let us illustrate the situation schematically by a further example taken from our treasury of trifles. In a conference room arranged for a forthcoming meeting the first participant has just made his entrance and walks around a long rectangular table to find the place reserved for him. While he is making his way, the view of the table changes, together with the optical-physiological patterns. The viewed is always the same; the sights are always different. Seen from the middle of a long side and from the middle of a short side the table presents itself in very different aspects. There is no position from which the four right angles are seen as such, i. e., in ortho-scopic projection, and yet from every position the table is perceived as a slab with four right angles and two pairs of parallel edges. The experience of "going around a table" is not limited to the awareness of the table. The observer moves, counteracting gravity in contraposition to a space resting in its own heft; the perspective aspects are not only grasped sequentially in relation to one another and to the "table" as object, they are also related to the changing positions of the observer; these once again are determined as moment-to-moment stopping points in the whole of the disposable space, which remains invariant while being traversed. In going around a table we follow—as always—a path step by step. When we do so our action is also determined by the relation of the part to the encompassing whole. For ages men have measured the length of a path by counting their steps. In walking the legs return after every step to their initial position, while the portion of the path being traced is always different. In walking, the walker's receptors are stimulated again and again at the same spot, namely at the soles of the feet, while, in his relation as part to the whole, he continually sets his foot on another spot on the ground [1]. We understand our own action of walking only then, when each single one of our steps refers, in antici-pation, to the next one and to the goal and retroactively, to those already executed and back to the starting point. The retroversion is no simple act of memory, in the sense of a reactivation of past impressions. I grasp the "whence" of my path in an inversion of the objective temporal order, just as in hearing and understanding a conversation we relate the last word of a sentence back to the first one. The accomplishment of inversion is directed toward the suchness and signification of the articulated sounds. The temporal order of the physical event of articulation remains unaltered. Only if and as long as we are able to separate the order of what is heard from the order of the hearing, can we, in the incessant flow of time, reverse the series A, B,

---

[1] The locus of optical excitation likewise remains always the same. The so-called exteroceptive, optical and tactile, stimuli are joined to the conventionally termed proprioceptive, stimuli. Out of such a melee of sensory data only a magician could construct the familiar everday world, which, in its elementary features, radically contradicts that primary "information". This demiurge would have to transform the succession of stimulations from the reflecting surfaces into the surfaces seen in juxtaposition; he would have to "project outward" the visual phenomena effected by optical stimuli, so that they would appear as the floor, evoking tactile phenomena; he would have to transform the phenomena already emerged into loci of future action; he would have to "project" outwards the visual data that arise in an observer's consciousness so that another person could tread on them. The mysteries of scientific positivism are peerless.

C into that of C, B, A, and thereby understand the passage of time and sequence in time as temporal sequence. The pointer of terrestial time, however, is set but in a single direction; it moves from a series of sounds, A, B, C to a series C, B, A no differently than it would move from A, B, C to D, E, F or from 1, 2, 3 to 4, 5, 6. The group C, B, A is the temporal inversion of the group A, B, C only insofar as *we* are able to perform the mirroring. A physical mirror of time does not exist.

Well, then, what holds all of these perspective views together and what holds them apart? „It just wouldn't make sense" if the view of the narrow side of the table should suddenly be attached to that of the long side. Evidently it is the table that unites, divides, and prescribes the perspective views and their sequence. It is the WHAT, the "sub-jectum" (in the original sense of the word), that persists as the same through all the separate views. In every moment we see *the* table; yet we never see it whole and complete, but always only in perspectival relation to ourselves. Language makes it possible for us to break through this linkage and to characterize the WHAT of the manifold views with one single word as one and the same.

Let us now assume that someone coming to the conference room has been stung by a tarantula, or that he arrives having had "one too many", or that he has just participated in a mescaline experiment, or that he finds himself in the preliminary stage of an epileptic seizure. What will be the result? How will our friend, who has just become our patient, see the room and table? We propose not to start from clinical experience, but to derive possible disturbances from the norm and then to compare them with clinical experience. It seems to me that one can distinguish the following phases of deformation, progressing from the milder ones to those more severe: 1. The milder disturbances of temporal inversion manifest themselves in the sensory asphasias, among others, in particular in those forms of pure word-deafness clinically differentiated as sub-cortical. 2. With the progressive impediment of the task of discriminating the bipolar order, we enter the zone of the so-called oriented twilight states. The patient, although still able to set his foot down correctly, is no longer able to apprehend diachronously the spot it occupies in the whole of the order of the Allon, and therewith his own coming and going. (To illustrate once more in terms of a card game: a tired player may still follow suit for the individual trick, but he may no longer be able to anticipate the course of the game as a whole or to reconstruct it.) 3. Successive views begin to blend. The long-sided appears shortened, the crooked straight, and the straight crooked. The views are neither entirely distinct nor completely integrated. They are no longer adumbrations of a WHAT manifesting itself as modified in a sequence. Firm shapes begin to dissolve in pulsating movements. 4. In the shifting of views the WHAT itself appears to be altered. The stability of visible things is dissolved—like a dream. 5. The disorder of the views is further aggravated by the patient's incapacity to determine his own position in relation to the surrounding whole. Thus the patient is helplessly exposed to a vortex of events. 6. Single views, following one another, no longer form a succession [1]. In this situation the patient would comport himself as a practicing nominalist; to him only—stimulus-bound—particulars remain accessible.

A single sense-datum, a single image, a single stimulus, can never enter into any kind of bond with another. The truly singular must remain entirely indeterminate. For each determination relates it to something else, which it borders and from which it is distinguished. As radically singular, a red spot cannot be grasped as red — for that would determine it in contrast to other colors; or as colored—for that would determine it in contrast to the tactile; or as a spot—for that would distinguish it from the surrounding ground; or as round—for that relates it to the angular. It could not appear "there", for that would be a place alongside and together with others; it could not be visible "now", for that would distinguish it from moments earlier or later. In short, we do not ascend from the singular to the encompassing and to the general; all determination is enacted in descent from an encompassing whole. We determine a point on a line, the line in a plane, the plane on a solid, the solid in encompassing space. In the same manner we determine an hour in the cycle of a day, a day in the cycle of a month, and a month in the cycle of a year. Finally, we determine our own existence in relation to the encompassing possibilities. Because we stand as parts in contraposition to the whole, we are able to determine the particular in descending from the whole. A sick person, unable to transcend any given point in time, and thereby to fit that moment into the total round of a day, must be incapable of comprehending morning, noon, and night, and to "take note of" what happened during a particular hour of the day.

It places no particularly great demands on our constructive-destructive phantasy to recognize in such disintegration of the I-Allon relationship the clinically familiar syndromes of the organic psychoses (disorientation, panic, euphoria, hallucinatory confusion, memory disturbances, twilight states). Also, phenomena known from experiments with mescaline, marijuana, and other drugs, like the intensification of colors and the optical destabilization, are easily comprehended, and the expansion of spaces and times, the experienced disintegration of the living body, are not too difficult to comprehend as manifestations of a shifting of the I-Allon boundaries.

With such considerations we have exceeded, after all, the limits of our theme. We had planned to let ourselves be guided by psychiatry to philosophical problems, and to try to solve these on our own account. We started

---

[1] MAYER-GROSS probably referred to such incoherence when he spoke of a "transitory interruption of the continuity of the psychic events".

from the fact that clinical experience requires us to investigate the hidden structure of the norm, whose disturbance is manifested in the comportment of the sick person. The application of the findings, if any, should be left to psychiatry. However, it was by no means our intention to launch from the secure base of the clinic a rocket that would briefly light up the nocturnal heavens of philosophy and then fade. In concluding we wish therefore to show that, and how, our presentation of the primary situation proves valid in an attempt to understand delusion.

Let us return once more to the theme of the clouding of consciousness as the axial syndrome of the organic psychoses. As mentioned before, the objections raised state—negatively—that a clouding of consciousness is not encountered in all phases of organic psychoses; they point—positively—to the delusional phenomena, which are said to be observed "with at least immediately maintained clarity of consciousness". This was also CONRAD's opinion, whose work I will once more use for critical comparison, since there are many points of contact, both descriptively and in terms of method. In his discussion of "apophany" (Apophänie), CONRAD offers a systematically elaborated sketch of normal comportment with the purpose of contrasting delusional phenomena against this standard. Delusional patients, according to CONRAD, are no longer capable of seeing themselves, as it were, from without, from above, detachedly, at a certain distance. They are incapable of performing the "Copernican" transformation, "which every healthy person can accomplish at any time". The "Ptolemaic" transformation is supposed to precede the "Copernican". In the clouding of consciousness the "Ptolemaic" transformation is said to fail, in delusion the "Copernican". Despite the fact that this second "transcendence" can succeed or fail only when the first has already been accomplished, it is CONRAD's opinion that in the paranoid hallucinatory psychoses the apophanic delusional experience can "become clouded". So the failure of the "Copernican" transformation is not conceptualized by CONRAD as a mere lack, it seems to me, since a positive content is ascribed to it, namely that of delusional formation.

CONRAD's theory of apophany is dominated by the traditional idea of the microcosm. Stepping out of himself in a transcendence "intentionally" achieved, the healthy person is said to discover himself as an "insignificant component" of a world common to himself and others. The relation to others and to the world is thus disclosed initially in a reflective act. The primary delusional formation is supposed to result from the disturbance of a reflection which the healthy person can and does engage in at any time. The "Copernican" transformation reveals to man his true situation. In transcending the bounds of microcosmic existence we realize that we are but a part of an immense whole and, relative to the many other human beings, just an insignificant part. According to CONRAD the accent lies not on the relation of the individual to the world, but on his relationship to his fellow men. In the "Copernican" transformation we learn our true worth, or actually un-worth, in seeing and measuring ourselves from without through the eyes of others. The end result of the "Copernican" transformation rests on an evaluative comparison.

One would think that with the failure of the "Copernican" transformation a painful insight would be spared us, so that we now, at one with ourselves, would find ourselves pleasantly well-proportioned. Delusions of grandeur rather than delusions of reference would seem to correspond to the failure of the "Copernican" transformation. In CONRAD's opinion, however, the "Copernican" transformation has the positive consequence that we step out of our egocentric position and thus no longer "relate everything to ourselves", while in failing to do so we live in the delusion that "everything revolves around us". Yet, it is not characteristic of delusions of reference that everything centers around the patient—for that happens to modern man as it did to the Roman conqueror; it happens to anyone who is at the center of society on a festive occasion. Rather it is characteristic of them that everything is directed at the patient in malevolence and that his enemies are masters to whom the patient is helplessly delivered up.

In our view, the discovery of being only a part is not due to secondary reflection; nor are we primarily a part in relation to other parts, but rather in relation to the whole, to the Allon. This relationship is not disclosed through ratiocination. With the rising up from the ground the relation of part to whole is immediately given; it is and remains the determining basic structure in all experiencing. The relation to the whole is directly experienced as an actual power relation; it is not posited by a judgment of value. Awake, we are able to secure distance from the Allon four ourselves in the bipolar order of experiencing, and to assert ourselves in contraposition to it. If in the whirl of events the stability of the Here dissolves, then the order of objects must dissolve at the same time. In the clouding of consciousness, i. e., when we are no longer able to fully assert our stand against the Allon, the intensity with which it strikes us grows. Objects lose their neutrality; figures in the wallpaper, for example, may be transformed into terrifying grimaces. The elementary physiognomic character of delusional experience already contradicts CONRAD's conception. CONRAD cites GRUHLE's formula of a "relationship posited for no reason at all". But nothing is *posited* in the paranoid-hallucinatory syndrome. The patient experiences the altered world in all its might. For that no other "reason" is needed than that of being stricken by a power that the patient is unable to disengage himself from. The mighty are not to be trifled with. Just as their word prevails, exactly as it has been said, uttered as a command that admits of no "ifs and buts", so too does the power of the physiognomic impression exclude every consideration of other possibilities. The world is not posited in judgment; it is not "believed" on the basis of experienced resistance (DILTHEY); it is neither "bracketed" (HUSSERL) nor unbracketed. Moreover, in psychosis it is not experienced as an objectively explorable order of things, as *ordo rerum*, ("re-ality") but as directly closing in, as "actu-ality".

In the clinical manifestations of the organic psychoses no new relationships are instituted. We are always under the impact of the Allon. Since it is a matter of principle that nothing radically new can appear in the destructions of the norm, the theoretical task of psychiatry is therefore accomplished only when the symptoms that surprise us in the clinic every day are rendered intelligible as possible destructions of the norm. Then we are able to understand the patients, even though we are unable to reach an understanding with them.

Whether schizophrenic delusions correspond to the paranoid hallucinatory delusional experiences of organic psychoses is a question that must first be considered and decided in the clinic. Thereafter the question may be raised whether and how the so-called endogenous psychoses can also be understood as forms of deterioration of the primary situation.

The title "Psychiatry and Philosophy" requires a full discussion of the *conditio humana*, so that insight into its structure will enable us to comprehend the destructions encountered on the ward. This enormous assignment cannot be accomplished within the framework of the present essay. To it both Psychoanalysis and Dasein-analysis have been devoted. In view of these endeavours and partially in contrast to them, I found it necessary to delineate first the "primary situation" common to man and animals, a situation from which the human world grows. Medical anthropology needs an anthropological propaedeutic.

Philosophy and Psychiatry

Maurice Natanson

"Philosophy", wrote R. G. COLLINGWOOD, "has this peculiarity, that reflection upon it is part of itself. The theory of poetry may or may not be of service to a poet—opinions on that question have differed—but it is not part of poetry. The theory of science and the theory of history are not parts of science and of history; if scientists and historians study these things, they study them not in their capacity as scientists or historians, but in their capacity as philosophers. But the theory of philosophy is itself a problem for philosophy; and not only a possible problem, but an inevitable problem, one which sooner or later it is bound to raise [1]." Any definition of philosophy, then, any effort to determine its proper scope and limits, any attempt to fix its essential task or locate its cardinal questions is itself a philosophic act and reflects, implicitly at least, some order of philosophic commitment. Philosophy is problematic to itself, and the philosopher is involved in a perennial struggle to illuminate the initial paradox of coming to terms with his own discipline. An historical approach to the traditional problems of philosophy is a science of beginnings, it is a radical attempt to re-view again and again the question of what it means to have a world, to be in a world, and to wonder about one's experience of a world. The triad of questioner, question, and the questioned may provide a clue to the unique dimension of philosophic concern.

As questioner, the philosopher confronts a reality that is not only problematic in so far as he, the philosopher, is a central and constitutive part of the "field" of his inquiry. For the philosopher is not just one among many objects in his world; he is a prime object, the condition for the possibility of there being objects at all. To be a questioner in reality is to locate oneself as part of the questionable and also as the source of questions. The questioner, then, may in a reflexive act recognize himself as questionable, as being part of the reality he seeks to comprehend. Raising a question, in this context, involves locating the world as capable of being questioned. A question presupposes what might be termed a fundamental dubiety; it emerges

---

[1] R. G. COLLINGWOOD: *An Essay on Philosophic Method*. Oxford: Oxford University Press 1933, pp. 1—2.

over and against a ground of what was hitherto taken for granted. In raising a question the philosophic questioner calls into focus for the first time the reality of the object *as* object, the nature of the given in experience *as* given. The questionable is the object of experience taken as "strange". As long as we live in the world within the mesh of its familiar lines, the object remains only potentially questionable. The philosophic act consists in the recognition of the potentiality of the object and the liberation of its presentative force.

More traditionally, philosophy is said to have two central functions: the analytic and the synthetic. The former attends to the analysis of basic terms, the clarification of meaning, the conceptual ordering of experience; the latter moves on to a view of reality as a whole, to an interpretation of the total scheme of things. Both are held to be integral to the development of a mature philosophical position. Taken together, they probe the fundamental nature of man's experience and provide a vantage point for explaining its signification. In these terms, the level of philosophical concern is not too difficult to locate: the philosopher is interested in a critical analysis of the fundamental presuppositions of human experience, in the sphere of common sense as well as of natural science. He is interested, then, in such structures as the existence of an external world, of fellow men within that world, of communication between men, of the dimensions of time constitutive of history and culture, and of the valuational character of human reality. Common sense and science are not essentially concerned with epistemology, with metaphysics; they commence where philosophers end. The philosopher locates as questionable what the rest of the world accepts as somehow obvious and certain. The philosopher, and with him philosophy, stands in a peculiar relationship not only to the world of daily life and of science but to the many disciplines that have historically been generated out of philosophical soil. In what sense then is a philosophy *of* science, a philosophy *of* art, a philosophy *of* history possible? How does philosophy stand with respect to its distinguished off-spring and relations? These questions cannot be explored here in their full depth, but it is possible to consider our inquiry into the relationship of philosophy and psychiatry as an approach, however tangential, to the problems at issue. Moreover, a consideration of the relationship of philosophy to psychiatry serves an immanent function: it again raises the question of what philosophy is, what its proper task should be. And in virtue of such considerations, another result may accrue: psychiatry may question itself in analogous fashion.

I. The Relationship between Philosophy and Psychiatry

There are two lines of development throughout the history of philosophy which have profound relevance for theoretical psychiatry. Before it is possible to explore the concrete questions involved in the relationship between philosophy and psychiatry, it is necessary to attend to a methodological distinction between the empirical-positivistic tradition and the conceptual-phenomenological approach to philosophical problems. The very expression of what one takes to be the relevant questions here will in good measure depend on the tradition in which the questions are formulated.

By an empirical-positivistic mode of philosophic analysis we may understand, briefly, a line of thought which places emphasis upon sensory knowledge, "hard" data, experience as the intersubjectively verifiable locus of man's action in a physical world. Negatively stated, empiricism stands opposed to the *a priori* determination of the nature of reality, and positivism defines itself, broadly, by its rejection of synthetic *a priori* knowledge and of necessary connection between matters of fact, and by its opposition to methodological procedures which are not based on the model of the natural sciences. By a conceptual-phenomenological tradition we would understand a decisive emphasis upon human reason, the ideational meaning-structure of experience, and a concern for the *a priori* and transcendental structures of human reality. Negatively expressed, conceptualism opposes radical nominalisms of any type, argues against the reduction of experience to sensory contents, objects to the rendering of mind as a passive receptacle into which experience drops its marks. Conceptualism commits itself to an opposition toward any view of experience which makes objects and events independent of mind, which considers the external world and its content to be structured apart from the constitutive activity of consciousness and spirit. Clearly, the history of philosophy may be understood as a dialectical interaction and evolution involving classical representatives of both camps, together with their related followers and intellectual descendants. It is impossible to trace out here even in outline the history of the developments involved, but it is possible to consider the contemporary situation in philosophy in so far as these traditional approaches find their analogues in the current scene.

The present dialectical tension in philosophy is between those thinkers influenced centrally by HUME, by the Darwinian revolution, by the rise of symbolic logic, by the new developments in physics and, at the other extreme, those historically molded by the Kantian, Bergsonian, and Husserlian tradition. Granted the unfairness implicit in all such dichotomies and reduction to "schools", it is still the case that a fundamental struggle is going on in present-day philosophy between camps which may not be united in themselves but which express essentially different concepts of Man. For the heirs of a naturalistically and positivistically oriented empiricism, Man is a being rooted in nature, in the organic and biologic universe that produced him. Concomitantly, the proper procedure for studying and understanding Man is, they claim, the utilization of a refined form of natural-scientific method. In this view Man is continuous with nature, and scientific method is eminently suited to the study of Man for the very same reasons that scientists have found it the surest guide to the uncovering of nature. It alone offers authentic intersubjective knowledge, it alone provides the basis for ultimately dominating the world. Contemporary naturalism, positivism, and other forms of empirically oriented positions are characterized by the fact that they hold, more or less explicitly, that the categories of natural science are sufficient and proper for the interpretation of the full range of human experience.

The descendants of the phenomenological tradition view Man in a more nearly transcendental frame. His mode of existence is not discontinuous with nature but is qualitatively different from that of the lower animals and the rest of nature. Whereas the inert objects of the world and lower animals are primarily *in* the world of their observers, the scientists, human beings are molders and shapers of their own reality; they possess a world defined by their ideas, their attitudes, their interpretive and evaluational schemas. In this horizon, consciousness is gifted with a quality that demarcates it from all other elements of nature: it is directly given to the human subject in the act of awareness. Objects and events are given *through* consciousness; they are not constitutive of consciousness. The task of a transcendentally oriented philosophy is the essential description of the real. Knowledge involves delineation and illumination but not, primarily, control or domination. Coming to terms with human experience requires *seeing* what there is, locating the categorial features of experience, and framing a systematic account of Man as a being who inquires into his own nature.

What follows now is an attempt to state the philosophic problems underlying theoretical psychiatry from the vantage point of the conceptual-phenomenological outlook. Rather than presenting either a comparison in depth or a dialogue between naturalism and phenomenology, we shall pursue the limits of a specific commitment, searching for the implications of one major way of seeing the world. It may be well then at the outset to characterize the phenomenological standpoint more closely.

Within every-day life, the "natural standpoint" in HUSSERL's language, we encounter objects, events, persons, and even ourselves, naively accepting all those already formed, epistemically shaped structures as familiar parts of our world. Common sense takes it for granted that there is an existent world, that each of us is in that world, that each of us is in it together with fellow men with whom we can communicate. Furthermore, we naively assume in every-day life that our world has a history, that it is an orderly affair which will, under normal circumstances, continue into the future indefinitely. Birth, aging, and death are equally familiar elements of the total pattern. In philosophic terminology, the mundane world does not know of the problems of an external world, intersubjectivity, temporality, or the metaphysics of death. Our very being in the world is, for the natural attitude, *our* being. And "world" as a philosophic concept lies on the far side of the ordinary imagination. Phenomenology is a radical effort to *review* all of these fundamental assumptions, and to gain access to a knowledge of what is given in experience apart from the pre-judgments and epistemic prejudices of a naive realism. The phenomenological task, then, is to examine what is given in its direct givenness, to turn to the essential features of what presents itself *as* it presents itself to consciousness, and, finally, to free consciousness of its root commitments by means of a procedure involving a methodologically radicalized doubt. Without going into the elaborate terminology developed in the history of the phenomenological movement, it is possible to turn immediately to the *kinds* of questions that manifest themselves in virtue of this style of philosophizing. More specifically, it is possible to see the order of questioning which philosophy addresses to psychiatry.

Let us begin with the level of daily life, mundane existence. The patient who confronts the psychiatrist in his office or in the clinic is a fellow man who appears, in a general way, to share the characteristic predicates of the genus Man; he is a psycho-physical unity, a being incarnate in the physical world. Apart from his mental or even physical condition, he is recognizable as a human being. The act of recognition, however, presupposes that the psychiatrist as observer confronts his fellow man within a situation that is itself part of his world. There being a world within which the encounter occurs is simply presupposed initially. The psychiatrist is not, *qua* psychiatrist, professionally interested in the question of the existence of the world within which his activities take place. Furthermore, he takes it for granted, philosophically, that if the patient is psychiatrically capable of communicating with him, communication itself is not a problem that falls within his province. Whatever the *problems* of communication may be, communication itself is unproblematic, i. e., the possibility of human beings being able to communicate with each other is taken for granted as "normal". Indeed, normalcy itself is largely a concept absorbed from our experience in the mundane world. Whatever the psychiatrist gains in understanding normalcy as a professional problem, i. e., as a central term of psychiatric discourse, he presupposes the very articulation of experience into the modalities of "normal" and "abnormal". It is no proper part of his direct concern that human reality has inherent modes of organization and expression. It may be questionable whether a given act is normal or whether a specifiable situation reveals pathological factors, but "act" and "situation" are as taken for granted in their philosophic status as are "fellow man" and "behavior" itself. What then does it mean to inquire into the distinctively philosophic dimension of such terms and general concepts?

Let us restrict ourselves to the analysis of one exemplary term: "world". It has already been suggested that for the natural standpoint of daily life "world" as a basic term is fundamentally taken for granted, simply assumed in ordinary discourse. It is no less the case that "world" is a cardinal presupposition of much psychiatric discourse. What exists, no matter what it is, exists in the world. What takes place occurs within the world. Our placement of objects as well as persons is always in terms of polarities or scales whose essential measure is the world. Our existence as men is within the spatio-temporal limits of our world. But what does "world" signify in all these instances, in all these usages? It may be suggested immediately that rather than there being any translation for the central term, "world" is naively assumed as itself the basis for elucidating the meaning of all the objects and events that are included within its confines. "World", then, turns out to be a "primitive" term of discourse; it is assumed in explanation as intrinsically beyond the need of clarification. Unfortunately, this assumption has profound philosophical implications which render its naive employment conceptually dangerous. To point out the essentially unclarified status of the term is the first duty of the philosopher as well as the first philosophic act.

The distinctively philosophical problem of "world" concerns its very placement within experience, not merely its linguistic form. We are not speaking here of definition but of conceptual comprehension. "World" is a categorial term, and by a category we understand a concept of the widest generality. Our initial way of being in the world (at the common-sense level) is being *with-in* "world" as a container of experience. The "with-in" structure of experience is presupposed in all specific predications: for something to be, to have a character or quality of any order is for it to have such status *with-in* the "world" of shared experience. The individual implicitly locates himself and the rest of his world in directional fashion, i. e., as being oriented toward some end, some goal, some boundary line or limit. To be directed toward a goal of any order is to be horizonally situated. In these terms, "world" is the categorial term for all directional or horizonal experience; it helps to inform us of the significance of being "with-in" a situation, of being "with-in" human reality.

Even a quick glance at the term "world" is enough to make the point at issue here: the distinctively philosophic dimension of the term is its meaning-status. "World" appears within mundane reality, including the mundane reality of the psychiatrist, as an already structured, formed concept. For the philosopher "world" is an essentially problematic term of experience. Its illumination involves an inquiry into its very possibility. In this sense, it is important to point out the underlying similarity between Kantian and phenomenological thought. Both are concerned with a transcendental investigation of the conditions for the very possibility of experience. And both are essentially *a priori* disciplines: they inquire not into the status or nature of the object but rather into Man's knowledge of the object. The transcendental question looks to the epistemological conditions which make experience of such and such an order possible in general. Finally, to speak of an *a priori* discipline here means only to emphasize the logical and not the chronological conditions which antecede the event. The level of discourse here is throughout epistemological, and this in itself demarcates philosophy from natural science as well as from common sense.

It is now possible to state directly the maieutic questions that philosophy asks of psychiatry (the implicit questions that psychiatry seeks of philosophy), but our list must be severely restricted. What follows must be considered representative and not exhaustive. We shall limit ourselves to the statement of those questions which we consider central but which can at the same time be meaningfully approached within the limits of this paper. Each question will then be taken as a section-heading for more careful investigation.

1. What is the essential structure of the world of every-day life, understood as the origin and locus of the problems with which psychiatrists must deal?

2. What is the epistemic root for the concept of "normalcy", which psychiatry utilizes and builds upon?

3. How is it possible that human reality has as one of its major expressions the "abnormal", or more broadly, the "morbid"?

4. How is communication possible in the mundane world, in the "morbid" world, and between these worlds?

5. In what sense are the concepts of etiology and therapy rooted in naturalistic-empiricistic categories, and what would it mean to re-approach them phenomenologically?

These questions will, finally, lead us back to another encounter with the methodological problems with which we began.

II. Questions which Philosophy Directs to Psychiatry

1. The World of Every-Day Life

It is an essential feature of mundane existence that within it the philosophical problem of mundane existence never arises. Or to put it in terms we have discussed earlier, within daily life "world" is presupposed. It might appear then that philosophy and common sense are eternal strangers or that common sense contains no philosophical problems. Such is not the case. Rather, we must say that philosophy is implicit within mundane existence, that common sense may itself be considered as potentially the richest of objects for philosophical inspection. Indeed, this was the insight which led EDMUND HUSSERL, in the last phase of his thought, to the discovery of the concept of the *Lebenswelt*[1] and ALFRED SCHUTZ to an approach to the phenomenology of the natural attitude[2]. More broadly, the phenomenological point of view here stresses the necessity of rendering naive assumptions explicit, bringing fundamental presuppositions of experience to light, and so reflecting systematically and rigorously on what it means to exist as man together with fellow men in "our" common world.

To speak, as HUSSERL does, of the *Lebenswelt* is to turn to the prime reality of our immediate experience, the world of meaning as it directly presents itself to men in action. Within this sense of "world", the individual's concrete acts, *his* performances, *his* situation, *his* unique awareness, *his* reality is the initial domain of man's being in the world. In fact, "world" reveals itself as the individual person's world above all. There is a qualitative difference between *his* experience of an event and the sociologist's, statistician's, psychologist's, or psychiatrist's placement of events of that type within common-sense life. The *Lebenswelt* is that sector of mundane existence lived by the person in his uniqueness. The concrete texture of an individual life takes on significance precisely in *Lebenswelt* terms. And it is in those terms that we may perhaps locate the essential features of the every-day world with which the psychiatrist begins epistemologically and from which he implicitly secures the central terms with which he operates professionally.

If the *Lebenswelt* is the primary locus of the individual's life, then its essential quality, we may say, is its implicit familiarity. No training is needed, no special instruction is required for the individual to recognize his primordial world as *his*. A translation of this assertion into the first-person vantage point of the phenomenologist may prove helpful at this stage. *My* world, then, is given to me without scientific or philosophical mediation as being "originarily" *mine*. And there is nothing tautological about this way of describing the situation. Rather, what is at issue is an interior horizon of experience through which each event in "my" world displays its characteristic texture. My way of arising, my way of bathing, dressing, eating, and going about the business of the day presupposes an unstated, even unformulated, purely implicit mode of recognition by means of which I greet each particular of my world as being indeed "mine". I distinguish, then, between the typical as I know it for others and the typical for me. And if I act in a manner which I deem to be almost

---

[1] EDMUND HUSSERL: *Die Krisis der europäischen Wissenschaften und die transzendentale Phänomonologie* (herausgegeben von WALTER BIEMEL). Haag: Martinus Nijhoff 1954, p. 105 ff.

[2] ALFRED SCHUTZ: *Der sinnhafte Aufbau der sozialen Welt*. Wien: Springer 1960 (zweite, unveränderte Auflage). English version: *The Phenomenology of the Social World* (translated by GEORGE WALSH and FREDERICK LEHNERT with an Introduction by GEORGE WALSH). Evanston: Northwestern University Press 1967.

identical in form to the acts of others, my act is nevertheless located within the horizon of my own immediately lived reality. A catalogue of all that is part of my world would include an endless list of particulars, but the listing would presuppose the relatedness of particulars to *my* sense of possession or acquisition. Thus I "have" my possessions in the mode of recognizing them as being infused with the essential quality of my being. Just as my shoes bear the specific marks formed by the shape of my foot and my way of walking, so each of my possessions is formed by the peculiar relation it bears to an informing consciousness. The possessions of my friend are familiar to me in quite another sense. I recognize them as tokens of a class, as typical exemplars of objects of various groups. But I realize that what makes my friend's possessions *his* is not that he has legal ownership of them but that their style of being for others emanates from the center of his defining attitude. If I envy my friend's possession of a special edition of a certain book, I may acquire a completely comparable copy, and yet my copy may lack the fascination of his. The special attraction his library has for me is largely explained by the aura of his home, his bookshelves, his way of handling his books, and not by the excellence of his taste or his bibliophilism. My envy in this instance stems from my awareness of the texture of an immediately structured world given unique valence by the particular human being who stands at its center.

In virtue of my "originary" grasp of familiarity I am capable of recognizing the unfamiliar, the strange. If the familiar may be understood as being grounded in the horizon of *my* world, the essentially strange may be interpreted as being fugitive from any horizon, as stemming from no one, as belonging to no person's world. Essential strangeness is clearly not synonymous with the unknown or the unusual. The latter are merely variations, expected variations of the familiar. Even if I have never seen a certain mammal before, I recognize it as a type of animal. Peculiar as it may be, it does not bear the menacing quality of the strange. Familiarity and strangeness, then, are not polarities of a qualitative unity; they are essential negations of each other. The horizon of familiarity establishes the limits of my world in its immediate givenness, whereas the strange irrupts in the familiar and transcends its outmost limits. Recognition of the familiar and the strange is a transcendental condition for the possibility of experience. It is based on neither inductive nor purely formal procedures; rather, the very formulation of a problem for inductive or deductive analysis takes for granted the location of the object to be studied. Recognition is an *a priori* of the *Lebenswelt*.

The scope of familiarity and the degrees of familiarity are problems of enormous complexity. My world includes a central, pervading milieu, but it also includes the phenomenon of the milieu of others; the concepts of routine, typification, the fundamental data of sleeping, waking, dreaming

are clearly parts of my world, as are the facts of social roles and of
sociality itself. It is impossible to attend to each of these thematic issues in
any detail within the limits of this paper. As a *modus operandi* we will
consider but one further aspect of the problem of familiarity as a structure
of the *Lebenswelt:* its intersubjective character.

The *Lebenswelt* is from the outset of my reflections your world as
well as mine; it is, in fact, *our* world. Whatever differences I recognize
between your style of existence and mine, I comprehend those differences
as demarcating a shared reality. My sensory awareness is personal or
individual, for the most part, in a relatively unimportant manner; what is
of significance is that my perceptual datum and yours point to or intend
the same object. Even perceptual life possesses a social dimension. Thus,
the *Lebenswelt* in being uniquely *mine* nevertheless reveals itself as
saturated with an intersubjective intent. *My* familiar world is in reality
inhabited directly or indirectly by fellow men and their activities. And
beyond my immediate social world there is the historical reality of the
past, the cultural dimension of the present, and the social expectation of
the future—our future. Language, morals, law, custom—all bear the
sedimented weight of a social reality which pervades the *Lebenswelt*. If
solipsism is a theoretical possibility, it is no less a practical impossibility.
For better or for worse, this remains *our* world.

It is from the *Lebenswelt*, then, that the psychiatric problems of the
individual emerge. The problem-laden patient enters the world of the
psychiatrist, the scientific observer, not as an object for inspection but as a
microcosm which reveals itself as both structured and structuring. The
problems that bring him to the psychiatrist's office or to the clinic have
emerged from the primordial world of lived experience, the *Lebenswelt*
of the patient and his fellow men. It must be remarked that the patient's
behavior, his style of being in the world, is first of all observed by
him and those concerned with him, not by expert analysts. The familiar
and the strange here manifest themselves in naive terms. What is taken
as "strange" behavior is "strange" within the horizon of our immediate
world, and it is intuitively encountered as extra-ordinary. The initial
discovery of mental abnormality takes place on the part of men within the
world of daily life. It is meaningful to suggest, then, that the essential
import of the phenomenological concept of the *Lebenswelt* for the psychiatrist is that it reveals the generic form of the "normal" and the root
meaning of its transformation into the morbid.

2. Normalcy

All discussions of normalcy in the present age bear the mark of
anthropological research: the central term is usually "cultural relativism".
It is proper to face this problem at the outset of our discussion. The

thesis of cultural relativism is that the normal is defined always by a particular ethnic group living at a particular historico-cultural period and has no necessary status, no ontological grounding, no bond to natural law of any order. The norm is relative to the time, place, and cultural matrix. It follows from this thesis that what is taken as normal in one society may be considered abnormal in another, that what is cherished as the highest ideal of one age may be considered despicable in the eyes of another. The end result of this line of reasoning is to deny the very possibility of universal and fixed norms.

Without entering into an analysis of the philosophical issues underlying the relativistic thesis, we may clarify our position with respect to it by first distinguishing between the form and the content of any norm. The latter refers to the specific claim made in the norm, the former points to the norm-character itself. Thus, the "what" of the norm undoubtedly varies historically and anthropologically, but the "that" of the norm is unchanging. It is universal for the human condition that men everywhere and at all times recognize *that* there is a course of action which is considered fitting and proper for certain situations. Indeed, the full range of social life involves throughout its structure a variety of normative conceptions of what is "usual", "fitting", and "right". There is no relativism involved in there being a normal course of action indicated for a vast domain of human choice and action. Claims about what the proper act should be in given situations vary, within a culture as well as between different cultures, but *that* something is expected as normal behavior is a constant of human experience.

In terms of the concept of the *Lebenswelt,* we may say that the particular values incorporated or realized within a given *Lebenswelt* may vary without the essential structure of the *Lebenswelt* being affected in any way. The "thatness" of the *Lebenswelt* reveals itself in manifold directions: human reality in its immediacy is a social reality, ego and alter ego are inescapable conditions for the social world. The sense of there being an every-day reality is an inescapable part of experience: the world is intended by consciousness *as world.* Thus, whatever the content of a *Lebenswelt,* its form is invariant. One may speak here of an "Ur-Lebenswelt" whose eidetic features constitute the ultimate ground for the meaning of normalcy, in so far as normalcy refers to "thatness" rather than "whatness".

The distinction just drawn between form and content serves another function. We are now in a position to see that the statistical concept of normalcy (the notion that our sense of what is normal is contingent on probabilities and averages) has no role to play in any interpretation of normalcy as a form-function. The "thatness" of the normal is presupposed in any statistical analysis of "what" is normal. "Thatness" is the phenomenological condition for the possibility of "whatness", and a direct inspection of experience within the *Lebenswelt* would help to clarify the "founding" relationship at issue. We shall forego such an analysis in favor of a more general account of the nature of the normal.

It was said earlier that both the familiar and the strange are primordially located within the *Lebenswelt* and that no expert knowledge is required for men in daily life to experience events as familiar or strange. An analogous situation pertains with respect to the normal. We perceive the world as normal in an originary act of seeing. And just as the familiar presupposed the horizon through which recognition operates, so the normal leads back epistemically to what we may term the horizon of typicality [1]. Objects, events, and persons are perceived not primarily as particulars but as universals, as typified forms. The child can never be taught to move from a mere given, repeated again and again, to the essential structure presented through the instances. Nor can he be taught to move conceptually from examples A, B, C, D, etc., to what they are examples of. The abstractive act is the condition for knowledge; it cannot, without moving in a vicious circle, be made the subject matter for instruction. But if we argue that initial knowledge is of universals and not of particulars, the impasse vanishes. Each object, then, is perceived implicitly as being object in general as well as being this dog or this tree. The type shines through the token. It is in virtue of the capacity to typify, the essential abstractive capacity of consciousness, that the *Lebenswelt* is experienced as normal.

The acts of typification are techniques of exclusion. In perceiving the universal and not merely the particular, consciousness "normalizes" its field of awareness by freeing itself of an extreme specificity and an overpowering generality. Excluded are the possibilities of lingering interminably over the given instance, of being caught, one might say, in its inward vortex, and also of being hurled outward in the quickening and expanding horizon of the general features of the given, its universal qualities. The type mediates between an utterly restricted and an absolutely unbound attention to the object of consciousness. If the first clogs the machinery of the mind, the second races its motor. Consciousness "normalizes" in the sense of freeing the particular from its particularity without eliminating its specificity. In equivalent terms, the universal is given limits which prohibit its conceptual acceleration. The normal is then a constitutive

---

[1] In the discussion of typification which follows we are indebted to the work of ALFRED SCHUTZ. In addition to the book cited above, see also his articles on "Common-Sense and Scientific Interpretation of Human Action", *Philosophy and Phenomenological Research*, Vol. XIV, 1953, pp. 1—37 and "Type and Eidos in HUSSERL's Late Philosophy", *Ibid.*, Vol. XX, 1959, pp. 147—165 (reprinted in the Collected Papers of ALFRED SCHUTZ, Vols. I and III. The Hague: Martinus Nijhoff 1962 and 1966).

feature of consciousness and not a compromise between extremes. Once again, we locate it as an *a priori* of the *Lebenswelt*.

The "normalizing" activity of consciousness directs itself to the form of what is taken as normal, not to its content. We are led back to the distinction between the "thatness" and "whatness" of experience. In these terms, the location of behavior as normal involves a transcension of particular contents in favor of an essential form. For example, we commonly recognize bizarre actions as "normal" if they come from a "normal" person. We consider an individual eccentric in his behavior if we consider him basically "normal". Radically peculiar acts depend for their evaluation on our estimate of the person who performs them. There are many styles of action which we recognize as "normal" possibilities for men despite the fact that they are markedly "abnormal" in themselves: drunkenness, fatigue, frenzy, melancholy, hysterical laughter, weeping, etc. In each of these instances we look to the performer, not his performance. We may conclude that "JOHN is not himself today", but we do not suggest that when JOHN *is* himself, it is in virtue of sobriety, vitality, calmness, etc. Seeing JOHN as normal amounts to seeing JOHN in his typical mode of being within the *Lebenswelt*.

The concept of typification has endless ramifications. It is in virtue of the abstractive capacity that the individual recognizes his placement within a social world which involves perspectives and roles, that he is able to come into contact, into communication with fellow men, that he is able to grasp his own action reflexively and consider its meaning in a rational manner. And, finally, it is because of the capacity to typify that the individual shares a common world with others. Normalcy, in these terms, is the essential capacity to typify actualized in human experience. The person who is bound by the particular or locates no limiting principle in the universal finds himself in an alien reality. He has been thrust out of *our* world into the aloneness of mental pathology. But he has not simply exchanged one world for another. To the contrary, he has given up central features of world as such. Although he may still be said to possess a world, it is more appropriate to say that he is possessed by a world. In any event, it is not the content of his new world that differs from the old, it is its very form. The qualitative movement from normalcy to disease involves a transformation of the world axis. It is the world itself which is rendered "strange". We may term the pathology of typification the "morbid".

3. The Morbid

If the essential capacity to typify is constitutive of normalcy, its breakdown or alteration in mental pathology displays itself in the transformation of the afflicted individual's world. A world-change underlies the specific alteration of his overt behavior. The radical illustration of such upheaval is the paradigm case of the psychotic. But it is unnecessary at this point to consider the full range of mental illness. What is at issue is the concept of the pathological itself, or, to use a somewhat outdated term, the morbid. What order of transformation creates the root-change in the psychotic's world? And how is it ontologically possible that human reality holds within it the possibility of the morbid? It is to these questions that the following considerations are addressed.

Contrast, to begin with, the case of the individual who is physically ill with that of the mental patient. The former shares our world, his troubles are confined to a segment of that world. Whether his case is light or desperate, it does not invade the totality of his being; he remains who he is despite the suffering or the anxiety he experiences in his illness. The mental patient suffers his disease in a qualitatively different way: the entire province of his being is affected, there may be nothing which does not or cannot bear the stamp of his disorder. It is the ordering principle of world as such that is affected in a radical way. It is easy to misunderstand the concept of order at this point. It is not being suggested that the psychotic's world lacks order; it is claimed instead that the informing principle for an ordered world has basically changed. An example may help.

Let us imagine a man who receives messages from a distant sphere which is not precisely a planet but an orb of special character which defies further description. These messages are transmitted to him by a process akin to a telepathy of the internal organs: certain intelligence is received by the heart, other information by the liver or stomach. The content of the messages cannot be translated into intersubjective form, but this is unnecessary because certain men are attuned to their meaning, and such men may be recognized by special characteristics which manifest themselves only on certain days and at certain magical places. It is unnecessary to carry the details out any further. Far from such a person lacking an ordered world, his world reeks with order: everything has connections, everything is bound to something else, everything has its proper translation, its interior and transcendent significance. What *is* lacking can be stated directly:

a) The *concept* of order escapes the person here: he cannot render what he experiences an object for his own inspection, he is unable to stand back and regard his own situation. Rather he *is* his situation.

b) There is an assignment of roles for others to play in the world just described. The orders are issued from a single source, and there can be no changes in the script.

c) The causal structure of the world is known only by the individual and can be translated through him alone. A sense of epistemic grandeur pervades the scene.

The "order" seemingly apparent in the magical world just described is in fact a pseudo order: it lacks an informing principle. That world is ordered which arises from the qualitative sense of order, from the "thatness" of order. And it is precisely a reflexive awareness of order *qua* order which is in principle denied the morbid mind. The change that results in the construction of a world is profound. The morbid world is never *our* world but simply world as it is. The subjunctive stance is ruled out. The architect of this world stands alone within it. *We* recognize him as strange. And what is strange is precisely the essential change we see in his world, not in the surface effects of performances. Earlier we said that the strange in its intrinsic character reveals itself within the *Lebenswelt* as emanating from no source. There is no contradiction involved. I do encounter the paradigmatic psychotic as strange, but it is not he who is strange. More strictly speaking, what is strange about him is that he is "not himself", he is another, a demonic possibility of his being. The ordering principle of his individuality has metamorphosed or vanished altogether. It becomes almost automatic to speak of a psychotic patient in the past tense: he was once a well-known lawyer, etc. The reference is not really temporal, i. e., we are not referring to the patient's former profession, we are implicitly asserting the disappearance of a dimension of his existence. A proper translation would be: "this patient when he was his normal self practiced law, but he is no longer that person". He is, then, someone with a double being: at once what he was and what replaced what he was. His world lies in the past waiting to be reclaimed.

The transformation of the principle of order into the strangeness of the morbid has an ontological dimension. Human reality reveals itself, as a matter of descriptive fact, in the modalities of the normal and the abnormal. The demonically strange is a central possibility of BEING. How are we to account for this? The comprehension of BEING involves two polar standpoints of explication: that of the actor and that of the observer. In "normal" experience each of us is both actor and observer of actions. We grasp the significance of our own action and interpret the acts of fellow men. Daily life is a dialectical movement between the thematic possibilities of self-interpretation and behavioral observation. Inherent within this dialectic, however, is the possibility of its disruption and severance into isolated sectors. From the egological standpoint which the phenomenologist employs, it is possible to say that my interpretation of the meaning of my own act eventually inserts itself in the world of my fellow man. They recognize me as a center from which meaningful action radiates. They presuppose that I interpret their action in analogous fashion. To separate one from the other, to reify it in itself, is to make possible a demonic mode of BEING. Each act my fellow man performs within the *Lebenswelt* is intended implicitly as a human act; it carries along with it the unsaid motto: this act comes from a human being. The BEING of the act is its intentional meaning-structure. To divest the act of its intended meaning is to locate an inverse mode of BEING. Similarly, my own interpretation of my own act has an intentional horizon of directedness toward others. To rob that act of its essential "sociality" is to reveal its morbid possibility. We see ourselves as well as others in terms of the integral perspectives of our *Lebenswelt;* when those perspectives are qualitatively altered or erased, the coherent elements of daily life are rendered strange. To consider such a transformation an ontological modality is to claim for any action or event a way of happening in the world. Normalcy and the morbid have their ontological style.

If the capacity to typify is the epistemological *a priori* of our common world of mundane existence, the implicit sociality of all human action may be said to be the ontological *a priori* of the *Lebenswelt.* That the world is *ours* as well as *mine* implies that a disconnection between the two would give rise to radically different ways of being in the world. The ontological dimension undergirds and transcends both the normal and the morbid because it is logically anterior to any order of valuation. Yet we do speak of the morbid as an inverse and demonic modality of BEING. These predicates are descriptive of *Lebenswelt* attitudes and reactions. It is interesting that medical science shares not only the same attitudes but takes them for granted in the same manner as do men in daily life. Health is superior to disease, and the overarching obligation and commitment of the physician is to heal. The root-choice involved here cannot and should not be explained or defended in terms of a particular ethic; what is at issue is an appraisal of ways of being in the world in terms of a direct encounter with the *Lebenswelt.* The decision in favor of therapy is a commitment to the intrinsic goodness of there being a social order, i. e., a community of men in living communication with each other. In this sense, psychiatry is an affirmation of the dialectical continuity between modes of BEING.

4. Communication

The existence of fellow men is an "ontological datum". The alter ego simply appears in the field of my awareness; I do not derive his existence from arguments of a theoretical order, nor can I "prove" his existence. Within the *Lebenswelt,* in Sartrean terms, the Other *looks at me*[1]. "Looking" and being "looked at" are phenomena rooted in "pre-predicative" experience; they presuppose a mode of being in the world which is anterior to reflexive analysis and to self-conscious inspection. Before I address the

---

[1] JEAN-PAUL SARTRE: *L'Être et le néant.* Paris: Gallimard 1943, p. 310 ff. English version: *Being and Nothingness* (translated with an Introduction by HAZEL E. BARNES), New York: Philosophical Library 1956, p. 252 ff.

Other, there is a zone of mutuality pre-predicatively given to "us": we confront each other in a situation which then permits the exchange of ideas. My fellow man is encountered as "within hailing range" or within "speaking distance", as available for an intimate chat, as open to a face to face encounter. In all of these possibilities, the Other is taken as "confront-able", as "hail-able", as essentially capable of approaching me in closer and closer relationships. He is already in the world moving toward me. Horizons of proximity and distance undergird the possibility of our meeting. The Other who is friendly toward me is said to be easily "approachable"; the Other who is rather cold, difficult to relate to, is spoken of as being "distant". The communicative zone involves avenues of withdrawal outward as well as engagement inward. To communicate is to be already involved in a world whose situations are built out of such eidetic possibilities.

To say of the *Lebenswelt* that it is above all an intersubjective world is to claim not only that communication takes place in it but that communication makes it possible. Within the "normal" world I can address the Other and expect to be addressed by him in turn. His *looking* at me promises his speaking to me, for the Other is not merely a body; as a person incarnate in the world his body is the instrument and the sheath of his mentality. The speech of the Other announces the bridge to his spirit, a way of crossing the zone of his objectness and exteriority and arriving at his person-hood. That there are levels of approach possible can hardly be denied. I may know the Other as friend or as lover, as acquaintance or as colleague, as stranger or as one of the mass of men. In each case, however, the horizons of distance and intimacy are dialectically operative. I may say of an individual that I once knew him well but have since lost "touch" with him, that I am coming to know him better and better, that I no longer "know" him at all, he has changed so radically. And it is clear that my communication with fellow men is limited by diverse regions of acquaintanceship: familial relationships, group connections, professional associations, sexual relationships, etc. Without attempting a positive typology of the manifold strata at issue here, it is possible to characterize certain central dimensions of all communication between fellow men within the *Lebenswelt*.

First, "normal" communication presupposes an on-going temporalization of address and response. The latter need not be verbal, but it must be intentive in nature and derive from a cognitive-emotive grasp of what was meant by the speaker. Superior monologues are restricted to the theatrical stage. In every-day life we expect the Other to answer, to speak up, to interrupt. The temporal order underlying the communicative act presupposes such interruption. But the mode of address need not be verbal either. There is, as GEORGE H. MEAD has pointed out, a "conversation of gestures". "Language", MEAD writes, "is a part of social behavior. There are an indefinite number of signs or symbols which may serve the purpose of what we term 'language'. We are reading the meaning of the conduct of other people when, perhaps, they are not aware of it. There is something that reveals to us what the purpose is—just the glance of an eye, the attitude of the body which leads to the response. The communication set up in this way between individuals may be very perfect. Conversation in gestures may be carried on which cannot be translated into articulate speech [1]". What is essential to the communicative act is that it binds ego and alter ego into a unit of expectancy dominated by a shared order of temporality.

A second major characteristic of communication within daily life involves the notion of so-called "interrupted activities". Imagine a conversation between men momentarily interrupted by the appearance of a third person. After the newcomer has been introduced by one of the group, the original conversation is taken up where it was temporarily dropped. "We were just speaking of ..." is a typical way in which the return is made to the theme which had been interrupted. All communication—and here we could go beyond face to face relationships and include correspondence, communication by way of third parties, etc.—is at bottom an activity destined in its very nature to be interrupted again and again. We might even speak of a conversation as an interruption between interruptions. The capacity to take up a topic of thought which has been discontinued is a crucial factor in all cognition. The individual is capable of communicating with a limited number of persons in face to face relationships; he must be able to suspend, break off, sever communicative action so that a larger order of social communication can be served. That human existence is necessarily structured into periods of waking and sleeping is deeply connected with the problem involved here. We might characterize man's being in the world as a perpetual movement within an invariant schema of interruptions.

Finally, it is a decisive characteristic of communication within the *Lebenswelt* that it presupposes a general clarity of mind and purpose, a consistency of intellect which makes possible both agreement and disagreement. Just as the Law of Contradiction undergirds the structure of logical discourse, so there is a Principle of Consistency which supports the communicative process. "Consistency" here does not mean mental discipline; it refers only to a unity of meaning without which "we" cannot talk to each other. Some of the conversations in *Alice in Wonderland* are instructive as well as amusing precisely because they are instances of the inversion of Consistency. Communication must necessarily have a subject term of discourse, and that subject term must be intersubjectively agreed upon. The

---

[1] George H. Mead: *Mind, Self and Society* (edited by Charles W. Morris). Chicago: University of Chicago Press 1934, pp. 13—14.

failure of the Principle of Consistency leads to the reduction of communication to the signs or artifacts that comprise its physical elements. One might imagine in adjacent cages two parrots trained to carry on what would otherwise be considered a rudimentary conversation. When the first parrot says "How are you?" the second parrot is cued to say "Just fine, thank you". Whatever else is involved here, communication is not.

In exploring the qualitative alteration of the communicative structure within mental pathology, we must distinguish between pathologic processes of language and speech and fundamental transformations of intersubjectivity. Language disturbances are often symptoms or products of organic and functional disorders; they are aspects of linguistic behavior within an inter-subjective world. The pathology of communication itself involves a different dimension of human reality. What is at issue here is the meaning of there being a world in which ego and alter ego share an experiential order in virtue of normalcy and lose that communality in mental morbidity. The psychotic's world can be understood but not shared. It is not possible to speak of patients psychiatrically classified in the same fashion sharing a world in virtue of their placement within the psychiatrist's typology. The situation is perhaps closer to the placement of the dreamer within his dream. Dreams are in principle solipsistic events. We attend to the reports of dreams; we cannot attend to the dreams directly unless they are our own. The aloneness of the dreamer is a phenomenological discovery, not a feature which waking life attributes to dreams as the upshot of a tautology. But it is the essence of dreaming that we awake after sleep and recall the dream. The psychotic waking state is analogous to the aloneness of the dreamer. Language is still accessible, conversation may be possible, but communality is gone. The dreamer and the dream cannot be distinguished.

How then is communication between the normal and the morbid worlds possible? The answer requires the rephrasing of the question. How is it possible for the normal man and the morbid man to understand each other? Since their worlds are structured in terms of radically different ordering principles, there must be the possibility of a principle of translation within certain limits. The psychiatrist translates the world-reports of his patient into the schema of the ideal-types and constructs which his discipline provides him with for the comprehension of mental disease. The patient lives within a world whose interpretive schema permits some translation of the behavior of others. The confrontation between men is transposed into the formal encounter between qualitatively different frames of reference and schemas of interpretation. The normal man is capable of rendering his schema an object for his own inspection and analysis; the morbid man cannot characterize his ordering principles, he can only express them through his naive behavior. The Other becomes dominant in the art of examination. The patient secretes the principles which might explain his being. In this sense, the morbid person is essentially secretive. His tragedy is that he possesses a secret he cannot in principle reveal. Exasperation with him is necessarily an improper response. One may be impatient with the man who knows but will not tell; it is unfitting to demand of the man incapable of telling that he transcend the limits of his condition. The remaining option for the investigator is the tangential procedure of endeavoring to relate the patient's world-order to the methodological constructs of psychiatry. Through a series of artificially generated typifications of morbid reality the psychiatrist attempts to comprehend the ordering principle of his patient's world, and so come to terms with the problems of treatment.

5. Etiology and Therapy

The category of causation is central not only to scientific explanation but also to scientific method. Most generally, science is concerned with establishing the order of events in nature, and this involves interpreting order as causal order. Explanation in this domain consists in setting forth with increasing accuracy the elements comprising events and placing those elements in concentric rings of increasing theoretical abstraction. To ask "why?", then, is to be properly answered in scientific dialogue by suggesting: "because of". It may be, as BERTRAND RUSSELL once said, that scientific procedure is founded on the fallacy of "affirming the consequent". Certainly medical science constantly faces the task of demonstrating that more is involved in therapy than can be explained on the grounds of *post hoc, ergo propter hoc*. The placement of cardinal emphasis on the causal structure of events is historically a deeply rooted aspect of modern science from the time of GALILEO to the immediate scene. The naturalistic tradition is committed to a causal viewing of phenomena because it claims that a true science, one involving adequate prediction and control, is possible only in terms of such a discipline. The model of physics continues to be the paradigm for the sciences, including the biological sciences.

A causal viewing of phenomena, however, presupposes that we are clear about the phenomena to begin with, i. e., that we have access to the events in question. Prior to the problems of establishing the etiological basis of a disease entity there is the problem of uncovering the phenomenal character of the disease in question. In the case of psychiatry, the disease entities are human realities expressed in the life activities of fellow men. Disease manifests itself within the *Lebenswelt* and is, as we have pointed out, originally recognized there not by experts but by ordinary men. The original response to pathological behavior is not through the question "Why is something wrong?" but "What is it that's wrong?" The "why" questions that follow are founded on the essential recognition *that* something is to be explained in terms that transcend the vocabulary of mundane life. If we follow the lead of human response at the naive level, we may come to an expression of a direct account of the phenomena of mental pathology.

At a more sophisticated level of analysis it is possible to distinguish between the causal-genetic approach to the morbid typical of the naturalistic tradition and the essentially descriptive attitude of phenomenology. The former views the event as a product, as the fruit of anterior circumstances and conditions; the latter sees the event in its direct givenness as having a status of its own, quite apart from what may have helped to shape or bring it about. In setting aside, methodologically, the question of causal relatedness, the phenomenologist is neither denying causation as a positive category of science nor refusing to examine its implications. Rather, the phenomenologist is attempting to "uncover" the phenomenon, to gain access to it apart from its already formed character within experience. The procedure of phenomenological reduction is completely misunderstood if it is taken to be a denial of the reality of the event or its causal connectedness within nature and social reality, its place in the world. Phenomenological doubt is an insistence on methodological neutrality. If the event is perceived in causal terms within the *Lebenswelt*, the phenomenologist will turn to the intentional structure of that perceiving, but he will do so in uncommitted terms. A non-causal examination of causation is then possible, and with it an epistemologically neutral inquiry into the status of phenomena in their causal relatedness to other phenomena[1]. In the phenomenological attitude, the problem of etiology is first the structural problem of seeing the elements comprising a disease entity in their elementhood. There is, then, a non-causal aspect underlying the concept of etiology.

A common feature of psychiatric practice is the desire of the patient to be appreciated in his uniqueness, not to have his complaints, his difficulties, his anxiety translated into typified causal terms. This is a desire that constitutes a paradox for the physician who does wish to see the patient as he is uniquely but who must, in the very nature of his professional obligations, proceed in terms of psychiatric generalization. A paradox within a paradox is generated: the problem of uniqueness replaces the unique person, and the former is itself typified. The formula: "Treat each person as a unique individual" contains its own refutation. A consistently naturalistic conception of etiology applied to mental disease faces a similar predicament. Whatever may be the etiological grounds of, phenomenologically speaking, my disturbance, I as patient have nothing to do with those grounds. They may be investigated by the observer; they

---

[1] MAURICE NATANSON: "Causation as a Structure of the *Lebenswelt*", *Journal of Existential Psychiatry*, Vol. I, 1960, pp. 346—366 (reprinted in his *Literature, Philosophy, and the Social Sciences: Essays in Existentialism and Phenomenology.* The Hague: Martinus Nijhoff 1962).

are distant from my situation. Such technical concepts as "case history", "environment", "heredity", etc., have no place within the limits of the *Lebenswelt*. The real challenge is to locate the individual in the texture of his immediately given reality as he lives it, and to reconstruct that world in its givenness without reducing its original features to alien categories. This is the task of a phenomenological *Verstehen;* it is the task of therapy as well.

A structural, descriptive orientation might appear to be pragmatically distant from the needs and concerns of the therapy-directed practitioner. In psychiatric practice therapy begins with the initial interview, it stems from the primary effort of the scientific observer to understand his patient. In short, therapy is an extension of the interpretive stance of the observer; it does not constitute an independent pragmatic dimension of medical practice. The central question here is not understanding versus therapy but rather what kind of understanding is required in the psychiatric situation. It has been suggested that a form of *Verstehen* characterizes the phenomenological standpoint with regard to therapy. This claim must now be examined more closely.

Verstehen, interpretive understanding, is an effort to comprehend the meaning an act has for the actor rather than the observer. Within the *Lebenswelt* the interpretation of world-events is first of all that of the acting subject, the ego who endows his world with meaning. The interpretive understanding of a fellow man's act must then be directed to the horizon of action as it articulates itself in the constitution of a world, the actor's world. Empathy is merely a fragmentary segment of a much larger pattern of concern. In interpretive understanding the investigator does not seek to place himself or imaginatively or emotively project himself into the world of the observed; rather, he seeks to grasp the signification of the action as it has original placement within the meaning-schema of the actor. The exploration of that schema in an individual case involves the effort, in principle, of reconstructing the eidetic features of a world. If the patient wishes to, seeks to be understood, that wish can be fulfilled in part at least by the effort the psychiatrist makes to *attend* to the patient's world. Creative listening on the part of the observer is an active participation in the "uncovering" of the world of the afflicted person. But listening in this context is not merely a matter of interviewing technique; it concerns the willingness of the physician to *see* the structural features of the patient's world *as* the latter livingly sees them. To regard them *as* the sufferer suffers them is not to suffer them oneself. *Verstehen* in this respect is quite divorced from empathic response. What is required of the psychiatrist is that he attend directly to the phenomena at issue. In a way, the implicit wish of the patient is that his world be seen in its integrity before it is altered. It must be seen in order for it to be transformed. What is at issue here is not just a matter of valuational neutraliy but of epistemic willingness on the part of the observer to *com-prehend* the structural features of an alien world. The phenomenologically concerned psychiatrist, then, must transcend empathy and realize that *seeing* is the first therapeutic act:

> "Take physic, pomp;
> Expose thyself to feel what wretches feel [1]."

The method of *Verstehen* as the clue to phenomenological sympathy goes beyond therapeutic technique in so far as it reveals an existential dimension. What GABRIEL MARCEL has termed "presence" and "availability" points to the intimate nexus between understanding and action. Both patient and psychiatrist are beings situated in relationship to each other as well as in relationship to the external world which, in one sense, contains them both. Coming to terms with their encounter in a segment of a more comprehensive world order involves an existential choice in which therapy is rooted. That is the choice of attempting to alter or transform a mode of being in the world. The structures of the *Lebenswelt*, the normal, the morbid, and of communication all presuppose that their elements are directly, livingly seen and grasped by man and fellow man. Without such structural *seeing*, therapeutics becomes a mode of rhetoric, an instrument of persuasion. And persuasion if it fails gives way to violence. When therapeutic violence fails, the right of the patient to his morbidity is acknowledged: nothing further can be "done" for him because nothing more can be done "to" him. Acknowledged failure then assures the accommodation of the patient in a special stratum of the social order. Lost to the *Lebenswelt*, he nevertheless secures a special status within it.

III. Methodological Afterword

The existential dimension in psychiatry, intimately linked as it is to phenomenology both historically and systematically, provides a vantage point for re-viewing some of the methodological problems with which we began. Whatever separates the wide range of existential thinkers, most of them are brought together thematically in their concern for the nature and status of the self in a reality defined by the categories of man's being in the world: his fear, dread, suffering, aloneness, and death. The human world is located by means of an inquiry into the structure and implications of such categories; the end result is a return to the *Lebenswelt* in a radically new dimension of understanding. If the *Lebenswelt* is the originarily

---

[1] *King Lear, Act* 111, Scene IV.

encountered world typified in normalcy, it might appear to be eminently distant from the reality described by existential writers, the reality of anguish, nausea, and death. Such a conclusion would miss both the meaning of existential philosophy and the nature of phenomenological description. A reappraisal of the *Lebenswelt* in terms of its existential dimension is necessary at this point.

Quite apart from moments of epiphany in which men in daily life see their world in depth, the every-day world is replete with qualities recognized as universally disintegrative: linguistic confusion, misunderstanding, failure, emotive inadequacy, unhappiness, disease, and death. Moreover, these elements are commonly grasped as invariant for the human condition: only the exceptional man escapes most of them. It is the manner in which these structures are recognized and acknowledged which brings the existential issue into focus. As KIERKEGAARD, HEIDEGGER, and SARTRE have shown, mundane existence is most often experienced within the "Aesthetic stage", in terms of "das Man", or through "mauvaise foi". The "uncovering" of the qualitative force of anguish, despair, and death requires a transcension of the "natural attitude", a rendering of the *Lebenswelt* as "strange". "Ivan Ilych's life", writes TOLSTOY in his famous story, "had been most simple and most ordinary and therefore most terrible [1]." MUNDANE existence is the the locus in which the self lives its life together with fellow men; its interior problem is how that self can achieve uniqueness when it is enmeshed in a typified reality. If intersubjectivity is the first characteristic of daily life, it is at the same time its deepest, most anguished problem. How is it possible for the individual to realize himself apart from others, and how is it possible for the individual to transcend the limits others impose upon him? What existential thinkers have termed the problem of "alienation" stems from an internal inconsistency in man's being and the being of the social order. SIMMEL has stated the case clearly:

"Society strives to be a whole, an organic unit of which the individuals must be mere members. Society asks of the individual that he employ all his strength in the service of the special function which he has to exercise as a member of it; that he so modify himself as to become the most suitable vehicle for this function. Yet the drive toward unity and wholeness that is characteristic of the individual himself rebels against this role. The individual strives to be rounded out in himself, not merely to help to round out society. He strives to develop his full capacities, irrespective of the shifts among them that the interest of society may ask of him. This conflict between the whole, which imposes the one-sidedness of partial function upon

---

[1] LEO TOLSTOY: *The Death of Ivan Ilych*. New York: New American Library 1960, p. 104. Cf. MARTIN HEIDEGGER: *Sein und Zeit*. Tübingen: Neomarius 1949, p. 254. English version: *Being and Time* (translated by JOHN MACQUARRIE and EDWARD ROBINSON), New York: Harper 1962, p. 298.

its elements, and the part, which itself strives to be a whole, is insoluble. No house can be built of houses, but only of specially formed stones; not tree can grow from trees, but only from differentiated cells [1]."

A typified world is then normal yet problematic for those who attend to it directly, i. e., who see the typical in its urgent and distressing texture. Such "seeing" is the gift of phenomenology and the point at which it merges with the existential tradition.

For HUSSERL, the root of the natural attitude is the "doxic" belief in the very being of the world. This is what HUSSERL terms the "general thesis" of the natural attitude. But this underlying, quite unconscious commitment to the reality of the *Lebenswelt*, we may say, bears a comforting suggestiveness: that our "animal faith" in reality is justified, that the typified world is as it appears to be, that we are then "safe" epistemically in an otherwise dangerous world. In short, typification as the central instrument of normalcy serves as insulation against the existential impact of *seeing* the world directly. Common sense, as ALFRED SCHUTZ has suggested, inverts the phenomenological procedure:

"Phenomenology has taught us the concept of phenomenological *epoché,* the suspension of our belief in the reality of the world as a device to overcome the natural attitude by radicalizing the Cartesian method of philosophical doubt. The suggestion may be ventured that man within the natural attitude also uses a specific *epoché,* of course quite another one than the phenomenologist. He does not suspend belief in the outer world and its objects, but on the contrary, he suspends doubt in its existence. What he puts in brackets is the doubt that the world and its objects might be otherwise than it appears to him. We propose to call this *epoché* the *epoché* of *the natural attitude* [2]."

Within the safety of not seeing the world, the existential categories are themselves grasped in merely socialized terms: "anguish" is a quantitative extension of unhappiness; "aloneness" is social isolation; "death" is what happens to others. The phenomenological investigation of the *Lebenswelt* places such "socialization" of categories in basic question, and it makes possible an encounter with the miracle of the ordinary, a theme more brilliantly developed in literature than in philosophy.

The location of the *Lebenswelt* as the root source of man's existence carries with it an existential-phenomenological character which is obscured and betrayed by the reduction of mundane existence to the data of natural scientific inspection. One may speak of the "mauvaise foi" of certain modes of the application of scientific method to human reality as well as the

---

[1] *The Sociology of Georg Simmel* (translated and edited by Kurt H. Wolff). Glencoe: The Free Press 1950, p. 59.

[2] ALFRED SCHUTZ: "On Multiple Realities", *Philosophy and Phenomenological Research,* Vol. V, 1945, pp. 550—551 (reprinted in his Collected Papers, Vol. I).

"bad faith" exhibited by men performing the "*epoché* of the natural attitude". The struggle for human authenticity at the personal level is matched at a more theoretical level in the encounter between representatives of the naturalistic and phenomenological traditions. What is at question is precisely the status of the *Lebenswelt*. It is the phenomenological position that the "data" of every-day life are qualitatively independent of the traditional schemas of mathematical physics and the scientific disciplines which attempt to translate the *Lebenswelt* into an extension of the material order. The impasse in contemporary psychology has been traced to the historical domination of physics. ARON GURWITSCH writes:

"Modern psychology has developed not only along, but also in continuity with, modern physics. What must be stressed is not primarily the definition of psychological concepts in analogy to concepts of physics. More important is the reference to physics in the very formulation of psychological problems, especially concerning perception. To explain perception, the psychologist accepts, and starts from, the universe as conceived in physical science, the true and scientifically valid universe. He also considers the human organism as a physical system acted upon by physical events. Independently of any theories to be advanced, the very problems meant to be solved by the theories, are determined by allowance for the science of physics. In this sense, both empiricistic and intellectualistic psychology has been dominated by what MERLEAU-PONTY calls 'le préjugé du monde'[1]."

Analogously, the situation in contemporary psychiatry has been deeply affected by the domination of a Galilean model of scientific explanation[2]. The cardinal challenge of the phenomenological approach to the philosophical problems underlying psychiatry is its insistence on conceiving man as a being in the world whose immediate life has a richness and validity of its own, a strength and a profundity which must be respected on their own terms. "Patient" and "psychiatrist" are abstractions from the world of lived experience: their encounter takes place within mundane life, and whether it is successful or disastrous, that encounter is a functional moment in the infra-scientific reality of the *Lebenswelt*.

---

[1] ARON GURWITSCH: *The Field of Consciousness.* Pittsburgh: Duquesne University Press 1964, p. 163 (cf. his "The Phenomenological and the Psychological Approach to Consciousness", *Philosophy and Phenomenological Research*, Vol. XV, 1955, pp. 303—319, reprinted in GURWITSCH's *Studies in Phenomenology and Psychology*. Evanston: Northwestern University Press 1966, and in *Essays in Phenomenology*, edited by MAURICE NATANSON. The Hague: Martinus Nijhoff 1966).

[2] See ERWIN W. STRAUS: *On Obsession: A Clinical and Methodological Study.* New York: Nervous and Mental Disease Monographs No. 73, 1948, p. 60.

Outline of an Organo-dynamic Conception of the Structure, Nosography, and Pathogenesis of Mental Diseases

Henri Ey

Introduction

A general doctrine totally "explaining" the object of a given science is impossible, and it can be said that even in physics no "theory" can be assimilated into such a doctrine but can only be a working hypothesis. The word 'doctrine', therefore, almost always and for each of us, signifies a pejorative judgment. In effect, it most often stands for speculation, abstraction, artificial construction, in short, ridiculous pretention instead of something useful.

Therefore in our domain, whose object—mental illness—is particularly difficult to conceptualize, it is impossible to be overly distrustful of improvised or too ambitious doctrines.

However if psychiatry wants to be presented and established as a science, it requires a conceptual system both clear enough and coherent enough so that the great problems which constitute the questions to which psychiatry must by definition respond can be presented, articulated and oriented, in such a way that they truly form a codification and an ordering of our knowledge. It is in this sense that KRONFELD (as BINSWANGER recalled some time ago) in his work *Das Wesen der psychiatrischen Erkenntnis* (1920) demanded that we leave behind the chaos of "heterologic" and "autologic" conceptions and constitute a more systematic and methodical pool of knowledge in psychiatry.

It is toward such a theoretical conception of psychiatry, or more exactly toward a fruitful 'working hypothesis' for theory research and practical application, that we are certainly all working, when, for each diagnostic or prognostic problem, for indications of therapeutic progress and in discussions of etiology or pathogenesis, the premises of a given theoretical concept determine our positions, and, consequently, our actions. Even the person who voluntarily declares himself the enemy of all doctrine must constantly, in each act of his profession, his art or his science, conform to some more or less systematic "idea" of the nature of the illness, the meaning of the symptoms and their evolution, etc. If, therefore, there is no general theory of psychiatry, it is not because it is better not to have one or because one must be content, in our discipline as in others, with a simple working hypothesis; it is because it is very difficult in this truly vertiginous area to arrive at clear and simple ideas without falling into the trap of over-simplification.

I. Preliminary Considerations for an Organo-dynamic Conception of Psychiatry

We can begin by recalling the words of CLAUDE BERNARD: "The time for doctrines and personal systems is past, and little by little they are being replaced by theories representing the actual state of the science and bringing to this point of view the contributions of everyone" (*Introduction à l'étude de la Médecine Expérimentale*, part III, chapter 4, paragraph 4). This time has also arrived for us, and we should be asking ourselves what lesson is to be learned from it. "Doctrines and personal systems" are less numerous in psychiatry than some would have us believe, for few works of our great classical thinkers and inspired predecessors have created doctrinal systems which have not been outmoded over the years. We should not, however, forget the doctrine of senile degeneration of MOREL and MAGNAN, the anatomophysiologic theories of WERNICKE, MEYNERT, and ZIEHEN. In contemporary psychiatry we can ponder the grand theoretical positions of PAWLOV, FREUD, JANET, JASPERS, BLEULER, KLEIST, MONAKOW, and MOURGUE, MINKOWSKI, BINSWANGER, GUIRAUD, SULLIVAN, etc. . . . What should we say with regard to these great systems, great ideas and great seekers when we suggest, in the spirit of CLAUDE BERNARD, that it would be better to replace them with a theory representing the actual state of our science and calling forth the continuing effort of everyone? We can only say: it is necessary to isolate from all these "personal" doctrines and too circumscribed theories a sort of basic principle or common denominator which will permit us to set forth with maximum clarity the science of psychiatry, to whose development so many authors have contributed.

It is therefore not necessary, in constructing this working hypothesis, to attempt originality. Neither is it a question of attempting to make an eclectic composite of the diverse tendencies and schools of thought which exist. It is rather a question of articulating and deepening the doctrinal aspects of psychiatry and then confronting them with the clinical aspects in attempting to achieve a coherent conceptualization which, being drawn from a great variety of theories, could coordinate the valuable and useful things that each of them contains.

It is "in all modesty" that I have driven myself for thirty years to accomplish this task, which is scarcely more than a matter of documentation, clinical observation, and reflection, without the merit of discovery and invention. In effect, I have never stopped searching for guides and allies for my own thinking, all the while putting aside anything which would be too personal or which would take me too far from the thinking of others. It is in this profound conformity of opinions, equally balanced by clinical experience, that I have undertaken this effort of critical synthesis which I would like now to discuss.

A scientific hypothesis must satisfy three major conditions before having some validity, especially if the hypothesis is to embrace so vast a subject as mental pathology. It must first be a verifiable codification of facts (from observation or experience); second, a coherent conception, both intelligible and transmissible; and third, of practical interest. Let us now discuss more precisely these unwritten laws, which should always be present in our minds.

The "empirical" aspect of a working hypothesis requires a strong clinical base. In other words, the ordering of our knowledge can only be founded on an extensive experience with the sick and the problems of diagnosis and prognosis which they create. One must, therefore, have spent a lifetime near these people in order to draw a maximum of benefit from the experiences of others. For this "material"—to use a horrible word—is the "empirical matter" which is the concern of the science of psychiatry.

The "logical" aspect of a theoretical concept requires that each part be integrated into a coherent system. This is generally considered by the theoreticians as the strong point of their methodology, while others consider it a major weakness. The theoretical concept must, then, develop out of a verifiable hypothesis on the structure and causality of the phenomena which are studied by psychiatric science. In this regard a *theory of the structure of the psyche,* whose pathologic variations we propose to present and reflect upon, becomes the fundamental difficulty which must be overcome by any logical approach to psychiatric problems. It is here that the science of psychiatry, in attempting to define itself, encounters its the greatest conceptual difficulties, inherent, really, in the principle of causality. Both causality and the solution of the mind-body problem are necessarily implicated in any psychiatric theory. Clearly, it is imperative both to be cognizant of the scale of the proposed enterprise and to be well acquainted with the discipline of reflection and the concepts of all those doctors, philosophers, neurophysiologists and psychologists who have deepened the study of man and his nature, culture, brain and thought.

The "heuristic" aspect of a theory, or rather its degree of practicality, requires more than a pure speculation without further interest. This is obviously even more true in psychiatry, a therapeutic science with numerous social repercussions. Some have believed that a theory, to be correct, has only to support an action which hopes to succeed. While this is not sufficient, it is at least necessary that a given theory have some practical corollaries. One could perhaps better say that more than implying practical conclusions, a theory must take into account the practical problems which are part of the definition of its concerns.

Because I believe this ideal of conceptualization can be approached in psychiatry, a science of psychiatry appears to me to be possible.

It is clear from what I have just said that the greatest difficulty is the question of a *basic hypothesis on the structure of the psyche*. This is the key to the success of our conceptual effort. In this regard, therefore, it is absolutely essential to question the traditional metaphysical positions which oppose each other and cancel out each other, i. e., dualism and monism. We must replace them with a pluralistic and hierarchical concept of the interrelationships between the physical and the moral.

On first looking at the problem we must avoid proposing a hypothesis based on "Cartesian dualism" (cf. my *Etudes*, Study No. 3, Tome I), for the opposition of mind and body, when *transferred to the psychiatric domain*, renders the idea of mental illness completely unintelligible. And such an idea must even necessarily disappear, either from being considered a cerebral accident indistinguishable from organic problems such as a tumor or a cerebral hemorrhage, or from being thought of as a "purely psychic" variation of ideas or feelings not unlike errors or sins. This, then, is the reason mental pathology has had so many difficulties in establishing itself, being squeezed, as it were, by this "psychiatricidal dilemma" (cf. my *Etudes* No. 1, 2, and 3). For the same reason physicians, philosophers, and theologians have been forced to speak in terms of a simple organic problem (i. e. phrenitis, etc., in Galen's time, or encephalitis at present) or a supernatural sickness *(Malleus maleficarum* during the Renaissance). From this same illusion of perspective come the battles which have exhausted the vitalists and the mechanists of the JACOBI-IDELER era and which still wander through the interminable discussions of today's psychogeneticists and organogeneticists. The point of departure, then, of our conception is that it can not and must not be inspired by sterile parallelistic dualism.

The other, or "monist", position is no better. For if dualism too radically separates the psychic from the organic, even to considering them as two heterogeneous substances whose causal interaction is unthinkable (except by using verbal artifice), monism, on the other hand, overmixes the two sides, reducing them to the same level and substance. Using the idealistic point of view of this monism it is impossible to identify and differentiate those mental illnesses which are comprehensible only when thought of as either the result of an eidetic vision or a hermeneutic interpretation of what is meaningful—in much the same manner as with other forms of human or natural beings. In the materialistic perspective of monism it is quite impossible to define the concerns of psychiatry because mental illness naturally assimilates mechanical phenomena and, really, the generality of things.

We are, therefore, going to follow a path which could be called "dialectic" or "dynamic" and which stresses the *movement which engenders the evolutionary passage from organic infrastructure to psychic superstructure*. This change in orientation is most important as it leads to a consideration of the *psyche* as a hierarchically organized structure rather than a juxtaposition of parallel essences (dualism) or as two sides of the same coin (monism). This old Aristotelian idea, which has been reworked many times by the neovitalists, psychologists, and philosophers (MAINE DE BIRAN, BERGSON, MAX SCHELER, KLAGES, NICOLAÏ HARTMANN, etc.), provides a good point of departure for our hypothesis. This idea permits us to bypass the sterile quarrels of both the ancients and moderns on psychic versus organic causation by making us return to the ideas of evolution *(Aufbau)* and dissolution *(Abbau)* both of which precisely postulate that mental illness is a *regression,* i. e., a disorganization of higher processes and a psychic reorganization at a lower level.

From a realistic point of view, therefore, we must take into account two fundamental facts.

The first is that *the psyche has a development*. It is impossible, after fifty years of study on the development of instincts (FREUD and the psychoanalysts), of intelligence (PIAGET), or of personality (PIERRE JANET, W. STERN, CH. BÜHLER) not to appreciate the successive stages through which the mind must pass to become adult—this long development from "infancy" to a man whose language and reasoning have evolved from the fragments and stumblings of the earliest life experiences.

The second fact is that man dreams when he sleeps. The psychic superstructure falls away leaving *a realm of the imaginary*. In other words, the psychic existence cannot be understood by thinking of it only as incorporating a *past* life (that of childhood) but rather as having an infrastructure, a *depth*. Put still another way, the structure of the psyche implies an internal organization, such that the actualities of experience meet the obscure and active forces which make up the unconscious. The being of a person is built on his first attempts at organization, always deep within the self. This is evident from the fact that when the conscious mind is unstructured during sleep or loses the power of self-organization as required by the demands of reason, it becomes prey to the unchained forces of the instincts and the imagination. One can say, in effect, that under the conscious mind which contains it lies or rather lives a level of unconscious virtualities, either past or passed by.

These two facts—one concerned with the *genetic perspective* (or "development"), the other with the *hierarchical perspective of psychic organization*—join together and complement each other in suggesting to us that the structure of the psyche is essentially *dynamic*. The relations between body and mind are neither those of contiguity nor of simple identity but rather dialectic relations involving evolution and organization. In this regard we can say that the psychic structure *constructs itself* just by moving from the level of corporal organization to that of a conscious mind and a personal existence. The more this construction progresses toward the psychic pole, the further it moves from the physical pole. So that we must substitute for the question of whether the genesis of a phenomenon is physical or psychic, the question: Is this phenomenon more or less psychic or physical? This really comes back to asking if it is progressive or regressive, normal or pathological. For to this idea that the psyche organizes itself by the progress of its evolution joins necessarily the idea that mental illness is the result of movement in the opposite direction (agenesis or regression).

Evolution *(Aufbau)* and dissolution *(Abbau)* would seem, then, to constitute the conceptual base for a working hypothesis in psychiatry, which is concerned with considering mental illness as a disorganization of the psyche.

Having come to this point of view, one naturally thinks of the work of HUGHLINGS JACKSON, the great English neurologist, as a sort of theoretical model. Undoubtedly his notion of evolution, progress and structural stratification of neural functions was borrowed from the evolutionism of Spencer. But even if this idea under its phylogenetic aspect seems—and is—problematical, the notion of a hierarchical ontogeny of the organization of the nervous system is still valuable and is sufficient. It has sufficed, in any case, for the neurological research of our time, as all the important works of PICK, HEAD, MONAKOW, SHERRINGTON, GOLDSTEIN, etc. were directly inspired by it. *The whole problem, therefore, is to determine if psychiatry can use this system of explanation.* As the work of JACKSON is almost exclusively concerned with the diseases of the nervous system and its various centers and functions, it could appear excessive and, in any case, risky, to attempt to apply to psychiatry a theory borrowed from JACKSON and conceived by him for its application to the "levels" of the nervous system. This reservation (or more exactly this prejudice) is often put forward by psychiatrists to whom—not without reason—the idea of purely and simply assimilating neurology into psychiatry is repugnant [1].

It would seem, then, that a fundamental revision of the Jacksonian concepts is necessary before they can be applied to mental illnesses. Apropos, JACKSON, in his famous dissertation on the "Elements of Madness" *(Croonian Lectures* of 1884) which one can find in *Selected Writings* (Vol.

---

[1] This can, I think, explain why, in the Anglo-Saxon countries, any attempt to apply the principles of JACKSON — meant only for the theory of nervous system diseases — to psychiatry (to the psychoses, especially the supposedly non-organic neuroses) is greeted with disdain. As if, for once, the Anglo-Saxons were setting themselves up as uncompromising Cartesians.

II, p. 411), suggests a solution to the problem of the relationship between neurology and psychiatry. In our first look at the possibility of *"The Application of the Principles of* JACKSON *to a dynamic conception of Neuropsychiatry"*, we emphasized (cf. especially in our commentary on JACKSON's text in note 7, p. 325—326, and what we wrote on this fundamental point in the conclusion of our article, p. 117—123), that it is necessary to distinguish between what JACKSON calls the *"local dissolutions"* of nervous system functions and the *"global or uniform dissolutions"* which correspond, according to him, to the various degrees of madness. This really comes back to saying that the notion of dissolution can only be applied in psychiatry to *"superior centers"*, in the realm of the integration of the psyche (as SHERRINGTON would have put it). And from this point, the validity of the application of JACKSON's principles to psychiatry depends on this question: In mental illness just where does dissolution apply? Clearly, in the neurological syndromes, the concept is well adapted to the functions and functional centers which anatomy and neurophysiology have described. But does it apply to psychiatry? Yes, according to the major hypothesis advanced above, which will be more explicitly discussed in the remainder of this exposé and which we can already formulate as follows: mental illnesses appear to be disorganizations of the psyche, and psychiatry is the science of these dissolutions (agenesis, disintegration, destructuration, regression, or other analogous concepts). But naturally this hypothesis must be validated, and it cannot be *unless, in effect, the notion of an organization of the psyche has an empirical foundation.*

There is the whole problem. If the answer is yes, there is no need to refuse to apply the general principles based on the ideas of evolution and dissolution to the area of psychiatry. If the answer is no, then all attempts in this direction are purely verbal and meaningless. We must, therefore, venture where JACKSON has not gone. For if I have sometimes called "neo-Jacksonian" the doctrinal perspective which I have tried to dissect out as a common denominator for the partial and confused theories of our time, I am in no way implying that I am an apologist for or a slave to the concepts of JACKSON. And here I repeat again what I have said so many times in my teaching and writing: the application to psychiatry of JACKSON's ideas *presupposes a revolution of Jacksonianism almost equal to that of psychiatry* (cf. my book *"La Conscience"*, Paris. P. U. F., 1968).

But even if the work of this famous English neurologist is enlightening and shows us in which direction to go, it is nevertheless not the only point of view capable of serving us as a guide and model.

In particular I have stressed many times the closeness JACKSON's thinking of the studies of MOREAU (de Tours) in his famous book on Hashish (apropos of facts which at present are being submitted to a great upsurge of interest in relation to "psychopharmacology"). Analogous ideas

can easily be found in certain German authors of the same period
(FRÉDÉRICK GROOS, ED. BENEDEK, HAINDORF, H. FEUCHTERSLEBEN and also
C. G. CARUS in many ways).

Still closer to us are the slightly out-of-date works of PAUL SOLLIER,
MIGNARD, and GRASSET, which are not without interest. They relate at
numerous points to the hierarchical conception of the psyche and its disorganization.

The French school of psychology and psychiatry was particularly ready
to welcome or develop thinking in this direction, having been for one
hundred and fifty years under the influence of the dynamist conceptions of
MAINE DE BIRAN and then BERGSON. It is remarkable that the work of
RIBOT, always inspired by the ideas of evolution and dissolution of psychic
functions, should have spread to all the psychologists and psychiatrists of
the end of the last century.

It is in the monumental work of PIERRE JANET that these theoretical
tendencies have found their most complete expression. His work brings
together two main sources of knowledge: 1. the experiments on hypnosis of
the French school at the end of the 19th century, and 2. the behaviorist or
pragmatist theories of the Anglo-Saxons (particularly those of WILLIAM
JAMES) on the psychosociological givens of primitive behavior and on "genetic" ideas in psychology (i. e., the notion of evolution and dissolution of
psychological functions). JANET's thinking integrated all the scattered ideas
at that time on automatism and on "psychological strength and weakness"
into a vast theory of the conscious mind and the personality, of the hierarchy
of reality functions and of degrees of psychological tension. Starting with
a psychological and quite clinical analysis of automation as a form
of disintegration of the conscious mind in hysterical patients, he
proposed a theory of the unconscious which implies that human action does
not involve superior levels or the full range of its voluntary, intelligent and
reality-adapted activity without first repressing primitive drives. For forty
or fifty years JANET worked to analyze the various clinical aspects of these
functional regressions that hypnosis, hysteria, and neurosis in general revealed by their destruction of superior levels of mental activity. At the end
of his life he applied these analyses to deliriums and hallucinations. Thirty
years ago I listened to him at the Collège de France. He took apart the
mechanisms of the actions of perception and memory; he dissected out the
anachronistic or regressive aspects of both feelings and behavior which
could no longer express themselves at the level of reality functions, and I
realized that here was the method, really almost a traditional approach,
that must be followed in order to arrive at a meaningful idea of mental
illness.

All that FREUD, with his methods, discovered—the *forces* of the unconscious, their dynamism, the conditions of their repression or emergence—all

this, to be encompassed by a psychiatric theory of neuroses, deliriums or schizophrenias, requires a theory of *psychological weakness* which would permit these forces to manifest themselves in the symptomatology of these illnesses.

Thus the work of PIERRE JANET, and above all the way in which it complements that of FREUD (an eventuality anticipated by many authors), acts as the foundation for a basic concept of psychiatry—along with JACKSON's neurological work. This conception postulates the fundamental ideas of the structural evolution of the psyche and its hierarchical organization at the various levels of the unconscious, the *"automatisme psychologique"* and the conscious mind—and their regression in mental illness. Such is, in my opinion, the sort of "common thread", present in the grand doctrinal conceptions of psychiatry, which ties together into one basic intuition JACKSON, JANET and FREUD.

In 20th century psychiatry other great works follow in this same path, and I will mention only a few of them. First the work of E. BLEULER. I believe that I have clearly shown the theoretical position of the "Master of Burghölzli" that enabled him to define the idea of schizophrenia. Essentially, his contribution consisted of pointing out the primary-negative-developmental aspect of schizophrenia on the one hand, versus the secondary-positive-psychodynamic aspect of the delirious, hallucinatory and catatonic phenomena of schizophrenic autism. In doing this he made an explicit application of the general series of ideas which I have just discussed, out of what had previously been merely a clinical intuition.

Secondly, we might consider the anticonceptual, antinosographical, concrete psychiatry of ADOLF MEYER as fitting into this theoretical movement, at least in its psychobiological aspect. Apropos, there is undoubtedly a theory in MEYER's work although he tried very hard not to have one (cf. especially the system of analysis and classification of facts, using the perspective of "ergasiology", which was regularly employed in the Phipps Clinic). The biodynamic theory of MASSERMAN also represents in a way an attempt at systematization using as a base the experimental research in this same doctrinal area. It is perhaps regrettable that Anglo-Saxon psychiatry (and A. MEYER himself) rejected any "theoretical construction" and could not be bothered with working in this particular theoretical framework. For if they had done so, they would have been spared the limited choice between a heavy, mechanical, "neurological" style psychiatry versus a too fluid, psychodynamic one.

H. CLAUDE, through his teaching between 1923 and 1935 (while inspired, as I well know, by the ideas of ADOLF MEYER and also those of BIRNBAUM) and through the dynamic orientation which he managed to give to his students' works (BOREL and GILBERT ROBIN, MONTASSUT, SCHIFF, CEILLIER, BARUK, HENRI EY, J. ROUART, etc.) created a school at Sainte

Anne which was inspired by the preoccupation of considering schizophrenia, the deliriums, hallucinations, and neuroses as functional disorders of psychic activity resulting from one basic organo-psychic condition.

KRETSCHMER, in his book on medical psychology, in his studies on hysteria, and in his systematic conception of the organization of the personality, has really taken an analogous position. One has only to read his pages devoted to the evolution and emancipation of hypoboulic or hyponoiac mechanisms in order to understand that his thinking is basically in line with our way of seeing things.

Certain other pivotal works of the last fifty years are also in this same theoretical "continuum". I could mention somewhat haphazardly the following as characteristic examples: the neurobiological concept of MONAKOW and MOURGUE; the remarkable analyses of perceptual problems by STEIN and MAYER-GROSS in the treatise of BUMKE; the articles of BRAUN, in that same work, on psychopathic reactions and personalities; the studies of STECK; those of J. DELAY (notably on the agnosias and memory problems).

It is not surprising, then, that when ROUART and I, in 1936, tried to discover in the work of JACKSON a kind of mother theory, at the same time H. F. HOFFMAN and MAX LEVIN were also trying to return to the principles of the theory of strata *(Schichte)* and levels of dissolution.

We can also mention, whether they refer to the same sources of inspiration or only imply them, the more recent works of K. CONRAD, BARAHONA FERNANDES, LLAVERO, and perhaps of BARUK on the catatonic state.

Thus the organodynamic conception of psychiatry has its noble titles. And even better, it can be perceived in most of the great works of psychiatry even when not playing a central role.

It is paradoxical, at the very least, that when contemporary manuals, treatises, or monographs delineate the doctrinal tendencies in psychiatry, they limit their discussion to a confrontation of organic versus psychogenic (psychodynamic) theories, as if, in effect, the organodynamic position did not exist. *It does however exist.* And it is necessary to those who misunderstand and combat it. As far as we are concerned, we believe that we have shown enough—and that is sufficient here to orient further development—so that based on the fundamental ideas of evolution, organization and hierarchical structuring of the psyche, the organodynamic position offers us a perspective which is perfectly justifiable by the convergence of ideas in such great minds.

If we designate this theoretical tendency as "organodynamic" it is to underline: 1. that mental illness is a form of disorganization in which the mental apparatus reorganizes itself at an inferior dynamic level. This is really postulating that disorganization, or if you prefer, *an organic sequence of regression*, constitutes the basis for mental illness—i. e., its negative aspect which, in the last analysis, defines and uniquely explains it; 2. that mental illness is always and necessarily a *dynamic structure*, a regressive form of consciousness or existence which is organized and exists at an inferior level, i. e., a level involving descent into the unconscious and imaginary mind. It is in such a way, let us repeat, that the model to which the mentally ill person necessarily refers us is the phenomenon of symbolic dream production by and during sleep.

For thirty years I have developed this organodynamic concept which, I repeat, is common to us all but must be further elaborated in order to be usable. Permit me, at this point, to mention the principal stages of this development. I began in my study on *The Notion of Automatism* what was finally put together, with ROUART, as a basic hypothesis related to the ideas of H. JACKSON (1936). Following this I discussed more explicitly the positions implied in the first approximation regarding the relation of neurology to psychiatry, and then the problem of psychogenesis.

The first three volumes of my *Etudes Psychiatriques* (1948—1954) constitute an attempt to synthesize psychiatry in this direction, and I particularly applied the organodynamic principles to the problem of the structuring and unstructuring of the conscious mind as regards crises and acute psychoses (Tome III of my *Etudes*, 1954). Since that time, I have exposed the organodynamic theses, in their various connections, in *Traité de Psychatrie de l'Encyclopédie Médico-Chirurgicale* (1955), and in my *Manuel de Psychiatrie* (1960). And I am continuing to prepare the next volumes of *Etudes* which will be devoted to chronic forms of mental illness, i. e., the pathology of the Person, his world and his reasoning (neuroses, schizophrenias, dementias and retardations). In other words I can only refer the reader who is interested in this attempt at doctrinal synthesis to the work I have done or am considering and to which references will be given at the end of this paper. I have not yet given up hoping to write the "Natural History of Madness"—encompassing both anthropology and natural science—that I and all psychiatrists have dreamed about.

Permit me, before undertaking as clear an exposition as possible of the essential points in the doctrinal positions whose synthesis forms the organodynamic conception of psychiatry, to say once again that it is only through this perspective that the structure, definition and theory of etiopathogenesis appear for what they are: *a pathology of freedom*. For to say that a man is "mentally" ill can only mean this: that he has fallen into the depths of himself—into this pit where consciousness turns to imagining, where his existence loses contact with reality, and where his personality is alienated and loses the equilibrium of reason. All these ideas stress the negative character of mental *illness* and the positive character of *madness* that is implied in all degrees and forms of affliction.

II. First Thesis (Psychological): Mental Illness is Implied in the Organization of the Psyche

The basic idea embodied in the thinking of JACKSON and the great neurologists who followed him (HEAD, SHERRINGTON, MONAKOW, etc.), and applied so appropriately to the disorders of the nervous system, is that "illness does not create but release" (in the sense of the German *frei-setzen*). The illness is not the effect of a mechanical sort of causality producing symptoms on a *tabula rasa*. Rather, disease disintegrates that which is integrated. Said another way, the *pathology* can only originate from a functional structuring or organization *(Aufbau)* which is characteristic of the *normal state*. When it is a question of "neurological" type illnesses (as I just referred to), one generally accepts this idea of an ontogenic evolution of nervous system functions in which one can recognize a true empirical content. And this reality is in large part objective and observable because it is nothing other than the structuring of the brain and nervous system. Embryology, experimental physiology, histopathology and the more recent discoveries of neurophysiology have all combined to give us an extensive, deep knowledge of this reality. It is so clearly shown that even the neurologists are reassured—they who never hesitate, for example, to consider aphasias, agnosias or pyramidal and extrapyramidal syndromes as system or functional center disintegrations. It is well known that the appearance of the primitive form of extension in the plantar reflex (Babinski sign) or the dissolutions of language at inferior levels of functioning in aphasia make up the prototypes for this theory.

But in psychiatry, things are quite different. I have already indicated above that this is what has pushed numerous authors to hold that the application of the principles of evolution *(Aufbau)* to the psyche was a purely theoretical matter with no real empirical content. And this is, as a rule, the type of criticism addressed to the concepts that we are defending here, by most authors such as GUIRAUD, BARUK, etc. And it is their complete right to be suspicious and to demand justifications and precisions. It is to this demand to be rigorous that the first thesis of our general hypothesis must reply.

In effect, it is a question of clearly demonstrating that *the development of the psyche and its organization* constitute a reality, and that the existence of a psyche assumes or presupposes a psychic organization. Perhaps HEYER is speaking along these lines when he mentions an *Organismus der Seele*, an old and basic idea that has remained in the minds of philosophers and physicians since ARISTOTLE and THOMAS AQUINAS. But one can understand that doctors, psychiatrists or neurologists would be quite sticky on this point, demanding enlightenment on "that which is dissolved", for they fear pure verbalism which would be satisfied with words only, *imagining* as many convincing examples as are necessary to "justify" the theory . . .

The empirical nature of our thinking must therefore be demonstrated— the reality of the ontogenic development of the psyche, if you prefer. And we must, at this juncture, recall to mind two absolutely essential groups of facts.

1. The Studies of Genetic Psychology on the Mental Development of the Child

We must take into account the following penetrating studies: a) On the history of the personality (W. STERN, CH. BÜHLER); b) On the organization of the personality and the integration of the primitive or archaic levels of reflex activity into progressively evolved forms (H. WALLON); c) On the evolution of self, this being formed, in its ascending movement, of repression of infantile drives and archaic concrete relations (FREUD and the psycho-analytic school); d) On the "operational gestaltization" of the types of knowledge and the construction of the reason (PIAGET). These well-known studies, which have furnished contemporary psychology with its true aims— the development of psychic life—Chapter I of our MANUEL—are there to show us that the psyche develops itself in successive phases which constitute the stages of its organization. The findings of *comparative psychology* (H. WERNER), such as the studies from ethnopsychology or zoopsychology, corroborate these facts by pointing out that in conditions where inferior social structures exist ("primitive"), the psyche remains fixed at *inferior levels of structuring which correspond to this degree of evolution*. And no one, I think, can say that this evolution is nothing. It must be said that it is really "something".

2. Studies on the Structural Stratification of the Psyche

These studies constitute one of the most striking aspects of modern psychology. They are saying, in effect, that if the psyche, during its development, passes the stages necessary for its organization, that these stages will remain permanently as a structural hierarchy of layers or levels *(Schichten)*. All this takes place as if the evolution through time remains as an infra-structure of the psychic organism. While the body, in the process of maturing, ceases to be an embryo, the embryonic development of the psyche remains virtually enveloped in the infrastructure of its adult organization. This hierarchical stratification is perhaps the most characteristic thing about the psyche, and that to which we will relate all the psychological aspects of the unconscious emotional drives of imagination, automatism and memory. One can even say that no description or phenomenology of psychic life is possible without introducing this dimension of "depth", i. e., ontological

regions which are the bedrock of being, its *Untergrund*. Whether by re-
minding us of FREUD and the virtuality of everything which is not actualized,
or by positing existence and the fact of a person being in the world (the
Dasein) as really the problem of a *struggle* for knowledge of self and
others against the "numinosus" of that which within man opposes his relations
with others—all psychologies, all modern philosophies, whether one calls
them *Tiefenpsychologie* (FREUD) or *"Existential analysis"* (HEIDEGGER),
or *"Structural psychology"* (KRUGER), etc., have unceasingly postulated the
existence in the depths of our being of the archaic layers of the instinctive,
fantasmic or mythical being. If certain authors or schools (FREUD, MAX
SCHELER, BERGSON, PALAGYI, PIERRE JANET, CASSIRER, GOLDSTEIN, NICOLAÏ
HARTMANN, G. EWALD, etc.) have resolutely placed themselves in this
perspective, it is precisely because it seemed to correspond well with
reality—or ontology of the psyche, if you prefer. In this regard, as I recalled above, the phenomenon of *sleepdream,* so central to the psychic life,
is there as if to remind us that *underneath* existence lies a dream, or what
comes to the same thing, that the *organization of the psyche contains the
elements of madness within itself.*

Also, the idea, or thesis if you prefer, that the progressive organization
and integration of the psyche is, in fact, a reality can no longer be doubted;
this idea is as clear as the certainty of the "cogito" or the existence of the
external world.

We can now describe in an empirical and concrete manner what should
be understood by *reality of the psyche,* a term which is not only open to
discussion but which asks a basic question preliminary to any application
of JACKSONIAN concepts to psychiatry.

To answer it, we must proceed with a structural analysis of the *conscious
mind* and the human *personality*. I was able to do this, while developing in
my own work the hypothesis whose dialectic framework is here being recon-
structed, by limiting myself to confirming it only by means of clinical experience—always the best way. I have, then, studied the acute psychoses
(Tome III of my *Etudes,* 1954) using as a *natural* starting point epilepsy,
states of confusion, borderline conditions, dreamlike states, and acute
delirious psychoses (which are often called *wahnhafte Zustände* and which
correspond in various degrees to the Latin *delirium). No less naturally,*
I have been led by events, really, to reestablish a continuum, lost for one
hundred years, between these states of confusion, dream-vision *(onirisme),*
depersonalization, delirious and hallucinatory experiences, and those conditions termed manic or melancholic. It took a great deal of reflection and
even courage to reestablish this traditionally broken link. But I finally went
ahead, under pressure from clinical requirements, and was led—I repeat,
quite naturally—to a grasp of the true structure of the conscious mind via
the clinical reality of its unstructuring. In effect, this conscious mind is

revealed to our gaze when we try to pull out and describe the psychic organization as the *synchronized* structure of the actuality of our experience *(Erlebnis)*. In this manner it defines itself as the organization of the field of consciousness in as much as this makes up the moment of our experience. At the termination of my clinical and phenomenological analyses, I therefore proposed the following definition of the conscious mind: "The conscious mind is that aspect of the psychic life which organizes all that has been experienced into a kind of representative awareness." Thus, the conscious mind is to the temporal what the body is to the spatial, an underpinning for our sensory experience. The phenomenological characteristics (i. e., the temporo-spatial structure of this "field", its horizon, perspectives and its constant movement between actual and extra-actual, between real and imaginary, between representation and perception, etc.) give this field of awareness an essentially dynamic form or *Gestalt* of the organization of the psychic life. But this *noxus* which brings alive within me the actuality of an experience through the "medium" of a living articulation with the world—this structure of the conscious mind—is a hierarchical structure. For the field of the actually lived is, itself, in constant and perpetual equilibrium with the underlying structures and forces of the unconscious. And any Gestaltization of this field implies an infinity of other undeveloped or hidden possibilities. On the other hand, this structure belongs to the body and has a substance. It is substantial in that it is incontestably linked to a cerebral function which constitutes the condition of its organization. It is striking to realize that the most recent studies in neurophysiology (MAGOUN, PENFIELD, etc.) are rediscovering JACKSON's initial intuitions on the role of the rhinencephalon, the old brain, and the limbic system, which are so tightly linked to the cerebral trunk in the stratified organization of the field of consciousness (Tome III, *Etude* No. 27).

Thus no one, it seems to me, can seriously argue that the basal organization of the psychic life or its hierarchical structure do not constitute a *reality,* guaranteed, at least in part, by its substance. Therefore the application of JACKSON's principles to this structure of the conscious mind is entirely justified—the example of epilepsy is a paradigm of it.

But we must go further still, for if the *field of consciousness* constitutes an ambiguous, objective-subjective reality where the experience and thinking which come from this reality are elaborated, it is then necessary to face this last problem: Is the *system of the personality,* "itself", capable of being reduced to phenomenological terms or of being structurally and genetically analyzed, and thereby capable of being submitted to this same principle of evolution (historical progress) and of integration (structural progress)?—without being mistaken either for a nervous system function (see KLEIST, for example) in neurological pathology as such or for the organization of the field of consciousness. It is undoubtedly true, in effect, that the "psychic being" or "Man" can constitute by themselves a *personality*—"psychic being" here defined as the "existing" *(Dasein)* which is the subject of its world and the object of the existential analyses of HEIDEGGER, BINSWANGER, and MIN-KOWSKI; and "Man" being defined in the certainty with which he can say that he is this "self" which I create by being myself in communication with an "other self". This concept—or more exactly this continuing existential reality of the true subject of all "cogito"—implies the other idea of an *autonomy of its reasoning,* to use the term which KANT employed to designate the supreme nature of being of this "moment of existence" *(Dasein).* The personality creates and constitutes itself as the affirmation of the self and as the subject of the world of self. It is in the individual specificity of this creation and liberty that man is the *Selbst-ich* of his own existence. All that is true, but the value system of the self (its theoretical and practical justification) has its own givens, plus a development, prehistory and history. It is not sufficient to comprehend man as a being who maintains only con-ditional and fundamental ties with the body and who surpasses this body to the extent of placing himself in the anthropologic space of co-existence in order to deny to this "Self" a "reality" which would only be given to objects. The "myself" exists but its specific way of being real is to be a construct whose progress is capable of being hindered or even reversed.

In effect, if one studies the constitution of "self"—as the authors whose well-known observations and analyses we have recalled above have done (P. JANET, FREUD, STERN, PIAGET, MONNIER, etc.)—one perceives quite easily that an integrative organization of the being of the subject corresponds to each stage of the development of aptitudes and the structuring of the conscious mind. To have a "diachronic" structure and to be essentially a narrative is, in effect, the true essence of this subject or "self". But it is also part of its essence to be a story which can be broken off or continued—in as much as there is an individual, or outmoded, existence. In this regard, the self must be the object, in psychology, of a longitudinal analysis of its being and becoming (or future). And it is really this organization or construc-tion of the self that the works I have just alluded to have most admirably demonstrated. This reality is obviously not that which would come to it from a space and an objectivity it transcends, but it is rather like a second degree reality, such as the second system of conditioning that PAVLOV himself was forced to introduce *over and above* his cerebral mechanism.

Let us now look at just how this "genetic" organization of the self pre-supposes the functioning of the stages or levels which go into its makeup. First of all, the self emerges as the *subject of its knowledge of the world,* and it constructs itself as a system of affective and logical values which individualize its existence relative to the common "reality", i. e., that concerning the legality of the reason. It is in this sense that the self is first of all the "logos" implicit in a verbal reality of which the use of the first person pronoun is the most concise and definite expression. In the early years of life, this original and basal construction of the self is linked to an apprenticeship to syntax and logic. Naturally, at this level, such a structural breakdown scarcely emerges from the neurobiological conditions which permit its first relations with others and the world of objects.

The second stage of development of the self corresponds to the problem of constructing its *world* insofar as it develops itself by elaborating "for itself" an image or representation of its world *(Weltanschauung)*. That is to say that it establishes a symbolic system of relationships (sentiments, beliefs) which permit it to face the social and natural worlds.

Following this, the "myself" is based on and develops within the problem of its identification as a *person*. This aspect comes about through the coherence and unification that the self introduces into its own personality as a sexual and social human being, having a vital and ideal program corresponding to its own way of identifying itself as being what it wants to be. And it is this structural level of the self that corresponds to its definition of social status and role.

Finally, the self is completed by becoming the *master of its own nature*. In assuring its own peculiar quality, it carries to the highest degree of differentiation all that contributes to a body and a temperament which are, in short, specific (while being, regarding temperament or biotype, part of the great variety of human beings). It thus gives to itself the physiognomy proper to its language, reactions and determinations [1].

This construction of the personality is accomplished, beginning with the cultural milieu and individual history, without, as I recalled above, the structure of the self (both actual and ideal) ever really breaking free, in its "ascetism" or "perfection of self", of either the original and historic determinations which in its memory cause to bear down upon it the past and its archaic infrastructures—or of the morphologic and energetic substratum which supplied its body. For on the one hand, the self is organized against all that within is *other*, just as the conscious mind is set against the forces of the unconscious; on the other hand, in the same way that the conscious mind is the result of the conditions of its substance, the building up of the self is the result of the totality of vital energies which are necessary to it.

Such is the psychological and anthropological thesis which constitutes our first theoretical position, which is borrowed from JACKSON but has been further elaborated as required by the interests of psychiatry. *Madness* (the

---

[1] Regarding this perspective, which is related to that of KLAGES or MAX SCHELER and also E. MOUNIER and which will make up my book *"Le Conscience"* and the next volumes of my *Etudes,* to be consecrated to the "reason" and the "person"—I propose thereby to reserve to ordering of the structure of the personality from the abusive way in which it has been introduced through the idea that a *Person* is identified by means of his biotype and character . . . (KRETSCHMER, EYSENCK, etc.).

alienation of self as the alteration of its emotional experience) *is implied in the dynamic structure of the conscious mind.* Mental illness—as we are going to see—is nothing other than the reverse image of this evolution. And this is the meaning we must give to the great thinking of JACKSON when he said that illness does not create but rather only "liberates" the infrastructures of being. Certainly this "liberation" is the opposite of liberty, since the disintegration of the psyche is its fall into the unconscious, imagining and archaic. Thus the domain of human liberty is guaranteed by the establishment of this first thesis opposing that of mental illness. The liberty of a normal man consists of pulling himself up from the depths and from the instinctive and automatic demands of his being. If one can say that all men are mad, this can only be in the sense that they all have within, like a pressing eventuality incorporated into the structure of their being, an urge toward the imaginary and unreal which they can only resist by the organization of their conscious mind and personality.

III. Second Thesis (Phenomenological): The Structure of Mental Illness is Essentially Negative or Regressive

G. CANGHILEM wrote in his famous work: *Essai sur quelques problèmes concernant le normal et le pathologique,* (1943): "Without the concepts of normal and pathological, the thought and activity of the physician are incomprehensible." And elsewhere (1951), he emphasized that psychiatrists are the physicians who have reflected the most on the problem of what is normal. And this is easy to understand. When it is a question of taking as the concern of pathology the "deviations from type" in a given species and for a given organism, the deviations are easy to observe, as the least of them is made into an illness. This is the case for organic afflictions which are made up of vitiations of vital functions and which involve a small margin of variation. Opposed to this situation, when we no longer consider man in his vitality but in his humanity, the individual as a psychic being is the center of an almost infinite number of variations and indefinite situations. To such a degree that the concept of "mental illness" has great difficulty—and has had for so many centuries!—in being distinguished from the mass of behavior variations, experiences, emotions or ideas by which each man has the power to differentiate himself from others or have personal and original contacts with others. This comes back to saying that the pathologic nature of mental illnesses, or really their definition, is not an easy quality to grasp as a psychiatric fact [1]. That a head cold or a bout of indigestion be called

---

[1] I have stressed many times, notably in my *Etude* No. 1 ("Madness and Human Values") that the appearance of the psychiatric phenomena of mental illness had coincided with the demands of problems created by the notion of individual liberty in modern western civilization.

an illness is not a very important or difficult medical problem, for it can
be resolved by its obvious nature and the small degree of practical importance of the question. On the other hand, whether a personality disturbance
or a state of anguish or jealousy is pathological or not constitutes a fundamental, practical and theoretical problem for psychiatry, which is both
difficult and urgent and which demands a solution.

Such is, in effect, the *requirement* of the definition of the pathological
nature of mental illness or psychic anomaly. Several years ago Dr. HEMMO
MÜLLER-SUUR dedicated a very interesting monograph to this important
problem (*Das psychisch Abnorme,* 1950). The whole empirical and logical
development of this idea is therein both clearly and rigorously set forth.
Even if his conclusions on the problem of the psychogenesis of the illness
and the ill person seem a bit too subtle or abstract, I will keep the essential
points (his conclusion is basically the same as that reached by Canghilem
in his analyses)—i. e., that the structure of psychic illness and the quality of
the psychically abnormal is incompatible with the simple notion of statistical
variation or deviation from the mean using a plain Gaussian curve. It is
this "qualitiy" which is now up for discussion and which we must now
consider in order to ask ourselves just what characterizes the structure of
mental illness.

At the outset it can be said that the classic mechanist dogma, which
developed in the shadow of Cartesian dualism [1], is presently untenable. The
mentally ill person—even the insane or demented person, as spoken of in
the perspective of the "heavy psychiatry" practiced in nineteenth century
asylums—is not a mechanical man whose afflicition would differ so
radically from the human condition that it could be defined as a collection
of symptoms mechanically produced or caused by certain lesions.

Let us say, in the opposite direction, that if we go now to the other end
of the scale of theoretical positions, we will find it impossible to follow
certain representatives (ever more numerous) of the "light psychiatry"
(Anglo-Saxon style) which is satisfied with defining mental illness as a
behavioral maladaption, a situational "maladjustment". This is like saying
that every individual who does not conform to the norm or the mean is
mentally ill—i. e., he who is *too* anguished, *too* moral, *too* perverse, or *too*
"passionate" . . .

If the first definition goes too far (illness as being mechanically produced),
the second (statistically abnormal reaction) does not say enough. The latter
is at least on the right side of the question, but the former goes far beyond
true mental illness, which is neither a simple personal variation nor a
mechanical monstrosity. Although mental illness could never be mistaken for

---

[1] cf. my *Etudes:* No. 1, "Madness and Human Values"; No. 3, "Mechanistic
Development of Psychiatry"; and No. 4, "The Notion of Mental Diseases and the
Place of Psychiatry in the Undertakings of Medical Science".

the viscissitudes, actions and choices of human existence, it can never be entirely freed from them. This is, I think, the conclusion that MÜLLER-SUUR comes to when he says that mental illness is a qualitative anomaly in the somatic dimension and a quantitative anomaly in the animist dimension. This is, it seems to me, like saying that sickness differs only quantitatively from the human condition while at the same time withdrawing qualitatively from it. It would be just as well to say that we find ourselves facing an ambiguous situation, but this ambiguity itself must lead us further towards attempting to comprehend the two fundamental aspects of mental illness as it exists: a) a modality of rupture in coexistence or communication; b) a true sickness of reality, i. e., sickness of the relationship of the "subject" with his world.

Said another way, in order to grasp mental illness in the "counter-sense" on which it is based, we must go back to the phenomenologic analyses of "intersubjective" relationships and of the *Dasein*.

1. Mental Illness as a Rupture of the Communication and Interrelationships Necessary for Comprehension

It has often been said (KURT SCHNEIDER) that the birth of the psycho-pathology of delusion *(Wahn)* goes back to 1913 and the famous work by KARL JASPERS. If this is so, one can say that the quasi-totality of the discussions, analyses, observations, and reflections on the structure of mental illness in general, constantly refers back to the applications of the principle of *comprehensibility* (of DROYSEN and DILTHEY) by that distinguished philosopher and clinician (JASPERS). Following this principle, there is reason to distinguish the point of view of *Verstehen* (to understand) from that of *Erklären* (to explain)—just as the pattern of causation in nature and science is distinguished from the sense and motives of the mind.

For fifty years there have been unceasing criticisms on this theme, and we cannot even think of exposing here the development of these innumerable discussions. In any case, it is sufficient to refer to that most lucid and well documented book of F. A. KEHRER—*Das Verstehen und Begreifen in der Psychiatrie* (1951) in order to have an idea of the substance of the controversies which erupted in the German-speaking countries (KRONFIELD, E. BLEULER, KURT SCHNEIDER, EWALD, K. KLEIST, C. BINSWANGER, ED, SPRANGER, MATUSSEK, KOLLE, etc.). In France the same problem and discussions began, following the work of CHARLES BLONDEL *(La Conscience Morbide—* 1914), between G. DUMAS, DE CLERAMBAULT, GUIRAUD, P. JANET, etc. These conversations reached a peak in recent years in that great discussion on the "Psychogenesis of the Neuroses and Psychoses" *(Journées de Bonneval,* 1957). Here, with J. LACAN and myself as the protagonists, the minds most representative of the young French school faced each other. Since that time the very lively discussions in *Evolution Psychiatrique* have prolonged the echoes of that confrontation. It is a question of nothing other than asking oneself if mental illness can be the object of a single hermeneutic approach, i. e., if sense and intentions are the *ultima ratio* of illness. Certainly a normal man is incompletely "clear" and understandable for other people in his ideas, conversation and behavior; and he is this way as much if not more for himself. As I have underlined above, the structure of what exists is essentially contradictory and conflicting in such a way that it hides part of itself from itself, and it fights what it doesn't want to be. For the "for-self" is a constant struggle between being and nothingness. Also there are a thousand reasons for saying that the criteria of intelligibility *(begreiflich)* or comprehensibility *(verstehbar)* cannot be absolute.

We can bring to mind so many things: the old discussions from the time of LEURET and FALRET; MOREAU DE TOURS on the diagnostic differences between the delirious idea and a simple error; the analyses of SERIEUX and CAPGRAS on delirious interpretations; the polemics between DE CLERAMBEAU and the school of CLAUDE on the meaning and motivation of hallucination; and more recently the divergent opinions of KURT SCHNEIDER, GRUHLE, KRANZ, PAULEIKOFF, MATUSSEK, and KOLLE on the affirmation or negation of a fundamental problem of perception in the *Wahnwahrnehmung*. And in pondering all this we always find ourselves forced to reply in the enigmatic way of the Normand: "Yes"—for the delirious idea, the hallucination, the obsession, etc., do have something in common with the psychic phenomena of normal life—"and No"—for experience *(Erlebnis)* of the these false perceptions, beliefs and imaginings is quite heterogeneous compared to the normal psychic life. Say what you will: use and analyze all the modalities of "to understand", "to feel", "to penetrate", and "to grasp", or sentiments of empathy (SULLIVAN, COTTWALL and DYMOND), or of sympathy; appeal to intuition, the intellectual process, motivation, etc. [1]; dispute even the relationship between he who must understand and he who must be understood (whether he wants to or not). Regardless, the psycho-pathological facts reveal themselves to us only in and by the rupture of "intersubjective" communications.

This impenetrability, the relative but decisive incomprehensibility of morbid mental phenomena, is not the result of a point by point (really "analytical") comparison of normal phenomena and pathological symptoms, but rather of the "seizure" of the structural ensemble of the psychic life. Well, to this point of view, the meeting *(Begegnung)* of the rigidity and the typicality of a jealous delusion or an incipient schizophrenia, these are clinical realities—i. e., reveal themselves to the clinician only in *Einfühlung*—of this "something" which escapes any psychological interpenetration, this enigmatic quality which makes up the *Hintergrund* of all symptoms

---

[1] cf. notably the small book by KEHRER, pp. 13—24.

and provides the opaque atmosphere which gives them their quality of being symptoms and not just the effect of a particular or mutual incomprehension.

From there, the observer runs up against the formal structure of mental illnesses, against this "remainder" which is either the bringing of psychic phenomena into the field of consciousness or the placing of aberrant values into the system of the personality.

Let us take, for example, the case of a "man who sees an angel" (to use an illustration from KLEIST). Naturally there is such a gradation of infintesimal nuances between this "seeing an angel" and "praying to his guardian angel" that it can be said that this phenomenon is only the exaggeration of a normal experience, i. e., the imagination. The relating of this phenomenon to an anguished or ecstatic state of mind can be another valuable and even fortunate attempt to establish some fruitful connections in our understanding. In the same way we can link this angelic vision with the desire to return to a state of innocence or to the fantasy image of a lost object. But the unmasking, the artificiality as such of the phenomenon, and its introduction into the hierarchy of levels of the "real" (as P. JANET has said) are all excluded from this great reservoir of motivation and comprehensive interrelations—i. e., excluded are all those things which are clear to the clinician who has continually noted and connoted the symptomalogical aspects (hallucinations, obsessions, impulses, etc.) of what is experienced as being incongruous or the invasion of some heterogeneous and mysterious "something". To present itself as this deformation, this disorganization of the field of perception, this upsetting of structure and the time and areas of existence—all this is, in effect, the phenomenological essence of all that is contained in the conscious mind which has been "unstructured". Thus, for the symptomatology of the destructuring of the conscious mind, the inability to understand existing phenomena is due to the anomalous way in which they are introduced into actual experience. That is why KLEIST proposed that this whole group of acute or symptom-producing psychoses be characterized by the *heteronomous* nature of the interrelationships of comprehension.

But let us go now to the other end of psychiatry, into the domain of deliriums and neuroses. If "the man who sees an angel" is a "man who says he sees an angel", i. e., who is giving us a fantastic story, there again we could undoubtedly say that this crazy man resembles a poet, a surrealist, or simply ourselves when we invent wild stories. But where does this madness begin for him—a madness which is so obvious to everyone that it would be paradoxical to say that only a psychiatrist can comprehend it for what it is, i. e., something which does not fit in with our usual way of thinking. Certainly, there also, the artificiality of alienation only appears to us in the absolute existentialist position of a "counter-truth", and in the reversal accomplished in the reality system of the subject who, for example, could at the same time admit that in his conception of the world one can see an angel just as naturally as an object—this despite all that we can understand of latent meaning and unconscious needs in his story, and despite occasional breakthroughs that we can accomplish by cutting through the metaphors, mysteries, and enigmas of his symbolic language. Going back to our example in another structural and profoundly neurotic perspective of the organization of the person—if "seeing an angel" is now "believing one saw an angel" or "making believe that one has seen an angel" it is to the extent and only to the extent that our phenomenological analysis will reveal that it is impossible for the person not to identify himself with a saint, that the phenomenon will take its place for us in the morbidity of this demand or inescapable need.

Undoubtedly in these last instances (delusion of grandeur or hysterical neurosis) KLEIST and also up to a certain point (which precisely summarizes the problem) K. JASPERS both speak to us, one (KLEIST) of homonomy, the other of "interrelations of comprehension" with respect to the development of the personality. But these phenomena, no matter how well their conscious and above all unconscious psychological motivation is worked out, are no less important as clinical manifestations of a psychosis or neurosis, precisely in the sense that their "significance" is taken as the misinterpretation of existence and implies that coexistence with others has assumed a pathological form.

I cannot hope to develop here all that one can find so admirably described and marvelously analyzed in the published papers of MINKOWSKI, BINSWANGER, VON GEBSATTEL, STRAUS, KUHN, etc. It seems obvious to me that all of them finally reach this "wall of meaning" which is traversed by the mentally ill person, whether he be neurotic or paranoid. Clearly in these cases, the impenetrability is not as marked as in dream states or in schizophrenia, which is like a dream existence; but mental illness, always and in all places, is seen for what it is—a rupture of communication and, in the final analysis, *a form of regression*. And we should stress the word form as well as the word regression in order to emphasize that the essential aspect of psychopathological structure is to be "held" or "fixed" in the inferior forms of development of the psyche.

2. Mental Illness as the Unstructuring of Reality

Having established that mental illness cuts the patient off from his communication with others and the common experience, we must now envisage just how the sick psyche disturbs the whole system of reality testing.

Undoubtedly this can lead us to what will appear to be overly subtle, complicated and philosophical reflections. However, it appears to me to be inescapable if we want to penetrate down to the real structure of what are called psychic troubles. In effect—the "psychic pattern" being the organization in a person which sustains his system of relating to others and to the objective world and also regulates the problem of his reality relative to that of others—it is impossible to say anything meaningful about its disorganization unless one penetrates to the basis for its normal organization.

Let us therefore say that mental illness has a singular and specific structure which does not permit its assimilation into an organic disorder *senso strictu*. For example, to say that someone has pulmonary tuberculosis or a liver abscess is to affirm that by physical examination or other physiopathological investigations the physician can "render objective" or prove the reality of the illness. If certain functional or dysmetabolic disorders fall outside of this requirement, it is only in the theoretical hope that some day the problem will be made more obvious and specific.

While mental illnesses can and must be brought closer to this objective reality, empirical or organic, it is not in their biological aspects that one can discover their essence and true definition. If we speak in terms of a schizophrenia, an obsessional neurosis, a delirium or a melancholic state, we can never truly comprehend these forms of consciousness and pathological existence without putting aside, as it were (as in parenthesis), the etiopathogenic factors on which they are based and conditioned. Stated another way, we must turn to an enlarged and deepened *clinical* method of phenomenological analysis of their essential nature in order to define mental illness and its various forms. We see right away therefore that mental illness, by altering and alienating the psyche, will present clinically in such a way as to raise particular and dizzying problems on the question of reality precisely because it is a disease of reality.

Let us first look at just how this mental illness makes itself known to the conscious mind and existence of the patient. It will not be a question of merely noting, as for a cancer or a sciatica, that the subject "does not feel" the tumor or that on the contrary he has pain—in other words to ask ourselves just what is the diagnostic value, in the mind of the physician, of the symptom in relation to the lesion. It will above all be a question of grasping the import *for the sick person* of the reality of the disease. In other words, we are immediately led to assign to the anguish, delirium, obsession or bizarre behavior which make up the clinical picture, a position in relation to the patient, because in the last analysis it is by comparing these symptoms to his judgment, control and motivations that these problems are clarified. This comes back to saying that we are at the opposite pole from external or veterinary pathology—and are really in the anthropological center of pathology. Our mentally ill patients manifest mental diseases which are defined in large part by the false reality which the sick person attributes to or denies them.

Very often—it has even been said that this was the true test of
madness—the sick person ignores, does not recognize or denies his illness.
And we will perhaps have much more to say here about the reticence and
bad faith of the delirious alienated person (especially the paranoid) and
about the troubles and perplexity which are hidden behind certain patterns
of denial. But on the whole we can say that for these sick people, the
illness does not exist because it is *named* by them as such: i. e., "real"
supernatural apparitions, "real" chases by the police, "real" persecution by
the neighbors, etc. The reality of that which has been experienced is replaced
by the reality of the illness, and the sick person finds himself in and says he
is in the best of health. "I would have to be crazy", he says, "not to believe
that." Such is the case with a seriously alienated person who has truly
reversed the categories of reality in order to deny the accusation that he is
mad or sick.

Many other sick people (on occasion even some of the ones we have just
talked about approach this) are aware that they are mentally ill. Especially
in most of the neuroses, depressions, anxiety reactions, and a certain number
of schizophrenias, melancholias, manic states, states of confusion, dementias
(at least in the beginning stages)—all these types of patients complain that
their minds are troubled. And when they hear voices, or feel depersonalized,
pushed into something or forced to act and think in a certain way, their
symptoms seem to them to be a strange experience whose reality—inadequate when compared with common, everyday reality—disturbs them.

Finally others are plunged into such a state (confusion, dementia, terminal schizophrenia, etc.) that outside of a vague feeling (a vague "consciousness") that something is wrong, no real problem is raised for them as
to the reality or unreality of an illness. This problem is removed by the
total absence of the question or difficulty of what is real.

Thus regarding the importance of the characteristics of their problems,
our sick people take many diverse positions as to the reality of their
illness. And, "on the whole", we can say that many mental conditions
escape recognition by the sick.

We are now going to see that they escape recognition by many physicians!
Let us take the point of view of the observer.

Certain physicians and sometimes even—we would not like to say
often—some psychiatrists, when they are presented with a "collection of
symptoms" (or as is sometimes said, "syndromes") jump "beyond" these
symptoms to some anatomophysiologic process. For example, one hears
them saying, "This is no mental illness but is 'really' a brain tumor."—"This
isn't a neurosis, it's an endocrine problem." And one can go so far with this
as to sometimes unhesitatingly agree that mental illness does not exist because
it is "really" a brain disease. In other words, for these physicians—specialists
or not of mental diseases—mental illness does not exist. In their eyes, only

the organic diseases, which they can see, exist, are real and make up the pathologic reality. They therefore contend that one must turn away from the clinical picture of these afflictions, which is without interest and quite imaginary, "to get to the bottom of things", i. e., to the causative processes. This return "to the real things" of objective reality is certainly not the approach recommended by HUSSERL, who urges us to seize upon the *phenomena* of the psychic life in their very essence and not to be content to pass them by or to consider the way they appear to us as a negligible point. This denial of mental illness as a reality validated by phenomenological analysis is an error as great as the denial, by the alienated person, of his mental illness.

Others, still more numerous, take up the same mistake in an opposite sense, in placing mental illness—by waving a magic wand—into the system of cultural significances, interpersonal and intersubjective relationships which make up the fiber of human existence—in as much as it is a story which unfolds with others in a succession of events and circumstances. For these people, also, there is no such thing as mental illness, which would be, as they say, only a "maladjustment", a "reaction", or a maladaption to the vicissitudes and difficulties of life (SULLIVAN). Thus, in the antinosographist schools of thought, no pathological reality is recognized in the mental illnesses, and it is found quite satisfying to reject them into the *caput mortuum* of Kraeplinian entities. In such a manner that, obviously not being "entities", they therefore have no real physiognomy. This is false.

This something which hides the structure of mental illness from the eyes of both sick person and physician can only come from this very structure. One must really grasp it for what it is, namely, a *pathology of reality*. This is obvious to anyone who admits that the organization of the psyche is nothing other than the basic of the relationships which regulate or govern its reality system. So that any alteration of reality is liable to be obvious to the subject and not understood by the observer—above all if the latter forgets that the illness can consist of precisely this unstructuring of the psyche which plunges it "really" and completely into the unreality of the imaginary.

But let us investigate things more closely by imagining some of the eventualities of this fall into unreality and the imaginary—a fall which, because of the very structuring of the psyche, will have a tendency to be lived and thought of as "real", i. e., not pathological as far as the patient is concerned.

When, like one who dreams, the mentally ill person falls into an imagining of a dreamlike experience [1], what he is seeing is imaginary, but

---

[1] To whatever degree this is, as I have shown in Vol. 3 of my *Etudes* on "Structure et la Déstructuration de la Conscience" and my book *La Conscience*, Paris: P. U. F., 2e éd. 1968.

in a form of experience which avoids the question of reality, in such a way that the ill person, like the dreamer, is living through a nightmare having all the attributes of the only reality he can still give himself or imagine. In this instance, it is only on waking up that the sick person asks himself if he dreamed or whether he actually experienced a reality. The impression of unreality, which surrounds the whole delirious experience *(Erlebnis)* with an air of fantasy and artificiality, persists, as "off-set" from the horizon of his conscious mind, only during the delirious experience itself. The importance of this retrospective "bringing to mind" or of its impossibility is very great in the clinical situation as WYRSCH (1937) has admirably shown, and more recently K. CONRAD (1958), especially apropos of the acute schizophrenias and their subsequent organization into chronic forms.

But the fall into the imaginary can also take the form of imprisonment in the archaic and unconscious layers of the system of the person and his world, while the structure of the conscious mind remains normal. This is the case with most of the chronic neuroses and psychoses. In certain cases—those showing a deeper regression of the reasoning mind, such as the dementias and the schizophrenia with marked dissociation—an autistic or chaotic world is substituted for reality ,thus ending in both the patient and the dreamer all possibility of even presenting to himself the problem of reality. At this stage the sick person is indifferent to his condition and unconcerned about his illness. In the case of the paranoid schizophrenias or systematized delusions, which form the most authentic model of self-alienation, the system of contacts which binds the subject to his world—i. e., the laws which control his beliefs, his conception of the cosmos and his emotional ties with the world of others—this system, the "delusion" *(Wahn)*, is made possible by means of a scandal of logic which "turns around" all the values of reality to the point of making madness the only reason for the madman. And it is this reversal of values, or self-alienation, which is like a challenge hurled by the sick man at those who would consider him as such. Finally, in the neuroses, disorders in which artifice makes up a fundamental structural dimension (play the fool, exaggerate, believe oneself sick, make oneself afraid, etc. . . . .) the collapse of "reality functioning"—as P. JANET would say—although less apparent in this type of illness, is nevertheless quite real. And this is basically because the patient has lost the power to regulate within himself the equilibrium between his unconscious and hallucinatory forces on one hand, and the structuring of his real "person" on the other. This is why he appears to an observer to be torn apart by some inner conflict. This very ambiguity is like the clinical manifestation of the reality of this imaginary illness—whether the conflict be symbolically displaced, or whether it must be deciphered from its symbols, metaphors and images as FREUD saw so clearly, or whether it is experienced by the subject as a most horrible reality and by the physician as a most incredible fiction.

Hysteria, which has in many ways monopolized the physicians' discussions of the notion of reality or unreality (sham, play-acting, pure imagination), can be more suitably considered as a limited example of a more general problem which is posed by the whole spectrum of mental diseases (whether they be psychoses or neuroses). But in any case it lets us see clearly that a basic part of the structure of mental illness is being *a disease of reality* or really an "imaginary illness", or better, "an illness of the imaginary". It is this negative aspect, this tendency to destroy the real, which constitutes its reality. Such is the reality of this unreality . . .

But once again, to arrive at a good understanding of what mental illness really is, one must have a "pattern" of organization and development of the psyche to work with. This will show us that its disorganization abandons it to the imaginary, that degenerated state, by creating the illusion—as in a dream—of a "reality" which is like the negation of its negation.

We have shown in our discussion that the negative structure of mental illness—its regressive, symbolic and imaginary aspect—corresponds to the idea that JACKSON put forward when he spoke of the *negative troubles* of disease. Only, in the present state of psychopathology and phenomenology, we are able to give more force, more depth and more richness to this "mother idea" of every organo-dynamic conception of mental illness. For an organo-dynamic concept of psychiatry is a theory which aspires, in terms of the evolution and structural hierarchy of the psyche, to consider the mental illness as psychic *disorganization*, i. e., as the true disintegration of the reality of the patient.

IV. Third Thesis (Clinical): Mental Illnesses (Psychoses and Neuroses) are Typical Forms — by Their Dynamic Structure and Their Evolution — of Various Levels of Agenesis or Dissolution of Psychic Organization

We have already had occasion to stress that the "mentally ill" person can in no way be confused with his anatomophysiologic substratum, whether we have knowledge of it or only imagine it. The famous example of general paresis should remove any illusions on this point. For if it is true that the psychic physiognomy of syphilitic meningo-encephalitis is very characteristic, it is no less true that other clinical pictures are seen which are effects of this same process (especially depressive forms), and that the exuberant dementia with associated megalomania can also be a manifestation of other cerebral processes (general pseudo-paresis). Thus if we go back to the very root of the great illusion of anatomoclinical entities, it is easy to realize that the idea of linking the pathognomonic features of a mental illness to a specific etiologic process is untenable. It was, however, the great dream of nineteenth century psychiatry to cut up mental illnesses into "entities" and to imagine some causal process which would link the clinical state with the biological substratum in a unity as "simple" as that formed, for example, in specific infectious diseases, such as the bacillus of Nikolaier and tetanus. More than that, the entity "appeared more autonomous the purer it seemed to be", that is, the more it expressed an internal or genetic causality (phenotypical). We will come back to this point later on.

For the moment it will suffice to say—as K. CONRAD recently remarked (*Nervenarzt*, 20/XI—1959)—that this "Kraeplinian" nosography could not be maintained either in the mind of KRAEPLIN himself or in those of his successors. It is really impossible to blind oneself to the "transitional forms" of the various psychoses and neuroses and not to see one ill person pass through several of these "entities" in the course of his illness. It is difficult also to blind oneself to the point of refusing the evidence from a whole spectrum of "psychosyndromes" or clinical pictures of reputedly "endogenous" psychoses manifesting the action of a clearly determined process (encephalitis, cerebral atrophy, hormonal disease, genotypical factors, etc.). Undoubtedly, the mind of the psychiatrist who is fascinated by the nosographical "myth" can always fall into error by turning to the notions of "true" or "false" illness, or by holding forth on what is essential or accessory to the clinical picture or on the concepts of "the threshold" or "precipitating factors", etc. I think it necessary to see the facts as they are. And they are and show themselves to us in such a manner that it appears impossible, in the present state of our clinical experience, to recognize "entities" except as in the *ideas* of psychiatrists. The progression of these "ideas", i. e., their history and diverse systems of classification, have been admirably described in the monograph by W. DE BOOR (*Psychiatrische Systematik*, 1954), and we are able to pick out, from the contradictions in psychiatrists' minds, that the only constant remaining is that a certain order of characteristics (*Zuordnungsmodi*) distinguishes what we call mental illnesses and is the basis for their reality.

It is, in effect, impossible to say that mental illnesses do not exist just because they do not correspond to specific etiopathogenic entities. The investigation of our "second thesis" has, I think, permitted us to establish that things just are not that way. Clinical work imposes on us the obligation to comprehend, in their phenomenological reality, the pathological forms of consciousness and existence which are typical enough to be *clinical types*—as KAHLBAUM said, I believe, when speaking of the habitual types, *Habitualformen*, which are the concern of a clinically based mental pathology. What are these "types", and what is their nature and their principle of classification? Such are the problems whose solution we must seek only in the clinic itself.

First of all, when we are faced with a "case", we are at one of the poles of our encounter with the patient, and we "assemble" everything in this patient which "resembles" what we have observed in other sick people. And, naturally, the possibility of founding if not a science *(Wissenschaft)* at least some empirical knowledge *(Kennerschaft)* depends on the possibility of comprehending this *physiognomy* which compels recognition—as a typical "Gestaltization" or as "phenomenological order". Whether the observer be ESQUIROL, GRIESINGER, FALRET, KAHLBAUM, KRAEPLIN, or SEGLAS—or some less distinguished person from our number—this labor of the identification of certain symptomatological profiles or constellations is indispensable in establishing the diagnosis, prognosis and treatment, and (beyond the clinical situation) the etiopathogenic concept which comes out of the preceding studies.

In this way of looking at things, all mental illnesses seem to be "syndromes". It is useful to analyze this idea of syndrome because it implies at least three meanings as used in general pathology. The first is that the syndrome is a mosaic pattern of symptoms, a simple *collection* of complaints. The second meaning of "syndrome" (as, for example, in "icteric syndrome" or "red nucleus syndrome") implies that a certain number of symptoms *signify* by their correlation that certain functions are interrelated and that a certain synergy is revealed by their alterations—i. e., a relationship between the production and breakdown of biliary pigments, the process of hemolysis and the metabolic cycle of hemoglobin in icterus; or the relationship between cerebellar function and postural tone for the red nucleus syndrome. Thus in the mind of the physician, the idea of "syndrome" has been established, through association and analogy, as a system of "anatomophysiologic correlations" which reveal or give meaning to the symptoms that compose them. "Syndrome" also implies a third idea: that of a pathologic manifestation which can be the expression of diverse etiologic factors. Thus, icterus can be caused by a hepatitis, a gallstone, or cancer of the head of the pancreas—and the red nucleus syndrome can be precipitated by a tumor, an encephalitis, etc.

However, when this triple concept of "syndrome" is applied to psychiatry, it runs into a triple problem. The first difficulty—corresponding to the first meaning—is that one cannot call a simple collection of symptoms a hysterical neurosis or a delirious episode without artificially pulverizing the meaningful unity of the clinical picture. The second is that "psychopathological conditions" such as "schizophrenia", "obsessional neurosis" or "persecutional delirium" do not share a functional link such as one sees in organic pathology. And this is why German psychiatry has reserved the title *Psychosyndrome* (BLEULER) for patterns of the exogenous reaction type of BONHOEFFER, i. e., that the concept is only applicable to cases which are closely related to neurological pathology. The third problem comes from the fact that the generative organic process is not always so obvious, so that, at least in many cases, numerous psychiatrists do not acknowledge its existence and most of them distinguish two classes of psychosis: the symptomatic or "syndromic" psychoses and the endogenous psychoses.

The notion of a "simple syndrome", to which one would like to reduce a mental illness, ends up by dissolving mental illness and almost necessarily, therefore, by cutting the field of psychiatry in half (the syndromes or mental illnesses and ... everything else). I stress once again that this is characteristic of the German school of nosography, but one is constantly finding it in French psychiatry, as in the classic distinction between "acquired versus constitutional illness" (DUPRÉ, ACHILLE DELMAS), or between the "mental syndromes" of somatic afflictions and moral illnesses (BARUK).

In the final analysis, the ideas contained in the concept of syndrome can be applied to "mental illness" only if one has a clear idea of its very structure, as we have established by formulating and developing our second thesis. This structure eliminates the first—and most superficial—meaning of the syndrome concept. We will see, by further discussion of the etiopatho-genic problem, just what profit can be gained from the third idea, i. e., that concerning an indifference to the clinical aspect with regard to the etiologic process. For the moment we can be satisfied to say—using the second meaning of syndrome—that mental illness has a "syndromic" aspect in as much as it reveals an "organization of the psyche" to which we are necessar-ily referred, but that its distinctive quality is really in representing not only a simple functional synergy but also an *inferior level of psychic organization* (both of the conscious mind and the whole person). This last requires a structural dynamic and also its own evolution. Mental illness is a syndrome, but one which is a "form of experience" *(Erlebnis)*, an event *(Geschehen)* or a pathologic manner of "being in the world" *(Dasein)*. And it is because we have been able to give a meaning to these words—by establishing our preceding themes—that we can employ them in the defini-tion of mental illness which is the concern of the clinical thesis that we are delineating here.

Naturally this idea that "mental illnesses" are the "stepping-stones" of the involutional movement of the psyche *(Abbau)* only has value if it is the corollary of a theory of the development and structural hierarchy of psychic life in the way we have discussed above. For if it is not, it only leads to vain observations and pure verbal constructs.

Having thus linked the nosographical problem to what we said before on the organization of the psyche and the negative structure of mental illness, let us now stress the differences between this notion of "typical levels" of evolution in the psyche and the notion of "entities". To propose that "mental illnesses" (epilepsy, paranoia, schizophrenia, manic-depressive psychosis, hysteria, general paresis, etc.) are pure and distinct "entities" is the same as denying all the principles of classification. For each of these entities is precisely and by definition autonomous, and therefore can only be defined and based on the evil genius of chance. This, I think, is what can explain the "chaos" of nosographies and classifications which are the shame of our special field. This chaos—of which the table of contents of successive editions of the great KRAEPLIN are a disappointing example—consists of accumulating pell-mell all these "maladies" just as the chance of their lesion or the ingenuity of the etiologic hypothesis bring them to us. And there is no sort of reasoning or maximum limit of increase to prevent an infinite addition to their numbers (the nosography of KLEIST is an example of this). On the contrary, as soon as one introduces the idea of the organization of the psyche, a principle of classification is born—even if it is false!—and we have established that it is not. Said another way, the notion of structural levels of organization and evolution places us in a dynamic perspective which guarantees a certain order and unity among the diversity of morbid types.

At this point we are led to consider the old concept of "unit psychosis" which was believed to have been well buried since the time of ZELLER and NEUMANN. However it is again being found quite attractive by those minds which have been confused by the failure of a psychiatry of entities (LLOPIS, MENNINGER, etc.—cf. the recent reflections on this subject by H. J. WEITBRECHT and W. JANZARIK). Certainly, along with this last mentioned author, one can foresee its application only to *endogenous psychoses* (W. SCHIED). But the very idea that the diversity of types is leading us to a unifying genre such as the idea of "reactions" (more or less ranked or standardized) to various etiologic factors, ends up necessarily at a "system" which encloses the whole spectrum of neuroses and psychoses into a single whole. It is therefore a question of a concept which is at the same time useful but also dangerous, in the sense that it can appear to legitimize the indifference of psychiatrists (especially the Anglo-Saxons or the psychoanalysts) to any nosographic problem. In effect, to say that there is only one way of reacting at the psychopathological level and that the differing modalities of this reaction are only eventualities of little importance, is to sweep away the whole effort of clinical classification which is employed by so many excellent clinics. No, it is not true that the object of clinical psychiatry is an *Einheitspsychose*. But the *theoretical* model which we are making here for this concept or *Leitidee* (JANZARIK) has a very real and important value. It comes back to saying, in effect, that there is a certain unity in the disorganization of the psyche, whose many pathological variations are ordered in relation to the very idea of this disorganization. It is the notion itself which is suitable to a general psychopathology in so far as such an entity would attempt to grasp the laws governing the relationships, transitional forms and movement toward dissolution *(Abbau)* of the spectrum of disease types.

Since we have clarified, in relation to our previous theoretical propositions, in what way the problem of classification of types of morbidity is raised in psychiatry, we must now attempt to say something helpful which will both let us escape from chaos and also allow us to integrate therein all the classical work of classification which our predecessors so patiently and methodically established. In effect, it is at the present time as absurd to hold on to the notion of "entities" as it is to refuse to describe psychiatric "disease types" which alone can justify the practical rules of diagnosis, prognosis and plan of therapy which must be applied to these mental illnesses.

If you care to refer to my *Etude* No. 20 (Tome III), you can read the following, which is really the plan of what I hope to prove by my clinical labors—a Herculean task of which the design, I am ashamed to say, so obviously exceeds my capabilities:

1. A "classification" must be neither a pure enumeration nor simply nomenclature, with open limits. It must be systematic, i. e., include in the general concept of "mental illness" all the variations which enter into the comprehension and extension of this concept. It must therefore start with a correct definition of mental disease, and it must be as clear and simple as it is profound.

2. The "mental illness", as we have seen in our *Etude* No. 4, can be defined only as a *clinical physiognomy*, a typical form of evolution of troubles in the psychic life, having a particular structure which is conditioned by a somatic process—i. e., developmental arrest or dissolution of the psychological edifice.

3. There is, therefore, every reason for separating out, in the natural history of mental disease, a double perspective: one consisting of clinical types or "typical reactions" which define the psychoses (and neuroses) as elements in a *classification of mental illnesses,* the other being the somatic processes which engender them, giving a *classification of pathogenic processes.*

4. The classification of mental illnesses is naturally divided into two sides, just as is the psychic life: the *pathology of the field of the conscious mind* and the *pathology of the personality.* The field of consciousness is defined by the psychic activity which organizes the actuality of present experience, and *personality* is defined by the trajectory of the existential, logical and permanent values of the individual (beliefs, rational or moral principles, ideal of self, etc.), the self as a system of historical development and of construction of the whole person.

5. The pathology of the conscious mind is made up of levels of dissolution or unstructuring which compose its activity. The "types" of acute psychoses correspond to each of these levels of disintegration. Whether it is a question of manic-depressive crises, bursts of delirium or hallucination, states of dream-confusion, all these acute psychoses represent the spectre of decompensation or collapse of the conscious field: i. e., a series of structural levels typical of this undoing of the conscious mind.

6. *Chronic mental illnesses* are defined as pathology of the personality, whether they include the reality of the troubles of the conscious field—while expanding this into the area of the personality—or whether they organize these problems into a viable way of life. These pathological types (forms) of personality

presuppose a lowered reaction threshold to account for the blossoming and subsequent durable organization of crises or acute psychotic episodes.

We can reduce our classification into more simple terms by use of the following outline:

Pathology of the Field of Consciousness (Acute Psychoses)	Pathology of the Personality (Chronic Psychoses and Neuroses)
Manic-depressive episodes (crises)	Disequilibrium. Neuroses
Delirious and Hallucinatory Outbursts Dreamlike States oniroïdes	Chronic Delusion and Schizophrenia
Dream-confused Psychoses	Dementias

My whole volume devoted to the acute psychoses is an exposé of the mass of clinical, phenomenological, and physiopathological data which justify *with facts* this first part of the classification. In short, the acute psychoses are essentially characterized by levels of unstructuring of the conscious mind which reveal to us its hierarchical structure. All these acute crises and episodes—including those seen in the clinic for *epilepsy* (the key example of all psychopathology related to the concepts of Jackson) plus those of the *manic-depressive psychoses*—can be organized in relation to the destructuring movement of the field of consciousness which appears at this point, through the spectral analysis of its pathology, as the result of activities which regulate the actualization of what has been experienced and compose the temporo-spatial organization of immediate experience *hic et nunc*.

I can only refer the reader to this work where I believe to have developed in most of its ramifications and in spite of its formidable difficulties, the indispensable clinical demonstration. The object of my share of the work has been, notably, the reduction of both mania and melancholia to this pathology of the conscious mind which the ancient authors tried so hard—and not without difficulty—to exclude. My goal was thereby to reestablish the continuum between the superior temporo-ethical level of unstructuring of the conscious mind and the inferior level of the dream-confusion-decomposition of the same mind. Anyone can see that, in any case, the thesis that I am defending here is the result of a sustained clinical effort and not in any way merely a facile mental construction.

Consider the idea of dividing "mental illnesses" into two classes—which are not mutually exclusive, as is clearly shown by the clinical manifestations of schizophrenia and the dementias on the one hand, versus those of epilepsy and manic-depressive attacks on the other. The first class consists of structural forms of the *acute psychoses* (taking us back to the pathology of actual experience up to the point of its fall into the dream state), and the second includes the *neuroses and chronic psychoses* considered as personality disturbances (examples of agenesis or regression). In any case, the idea of such a division will be surprising only to those who are ignorant of the history of ideas in medicine or who refuse to understand that to say a man is chronically ill mentally, is to say that he is affected in the permanent organization of his being, i. e., in what really makes him a person.

It has already been a long time since SYDENHAM [1] first began the idea, in pathology, of the contrast between acute and chronic illness—not at all in the sense of curable versus incurable, but as conditions with a *cursus morbi* of quite different structure. The former (acute) are beneficial crises, vital catastrophies which do not alter the vitality of the sick person and may even protect him. The latter (chronic) are like a slow process during which the organism sets up within itself a diseased or pathological equilibrium—or homeostasis as we would now express it. Well, the pathology of the conscious mind represents, in the area of mental illness, this fall or plunge into the dream world which has a cathartic or reparative power. By contrast, the "chronic mental afflictions" are disorganizations of the psyche in as much as this psyche develops from this point in a completely different direction from that of the self *(Moi)*. Perhaps W. JANZARIK, in his just published work [2], has rediscovered the same intuition by attempting to discover these *dynamische Grundkonstellationen in endogenen Psychosen,* and by opposing the problems of "realization in the area of representation" to the *dynamische Geschehen.* And this is again the same idea that one finds in the book by K. CONRAD on *Die beginnende Schizophrenie.* I can put down here only a few indications of the direction of the work I am pursuing at present and which will make up the material of volumes yet to be written. Also I beg the reader to consider what now follows as only a beginning approximation.

By "chronic mental illnesses" I mean all types of psychological problems which come about by modifying the very system of the personality. Usually this occurs via a slow progression which terminates with a pathological equilibrium which is reversible only with great difficulty. Therefore all these mental illnesses—all the neuroses, chronic deliriums, schizophrenias and dementias—all are characterized by a dynamic unstructuring of the system of the personality. It certainly takes a great deal of courage to upset, by saying this, so many inherited and classical ideas and to "put in the same bag" the dementias and the neuroses—and I am leaving out, in the interests

---

[1] SYDENHAM, *Dissertatio epistolaris ad Guilielmum Cole,* cf. on this subject the profound study of LAÏN ENTRALGO: *La Historica Clinica,* Madrid, 1950.

[2] I was only able to begin reading it the same day I was writing these pages — a difficult task for one such as myself who reads German quite slowly.

of clarity, the problems of agenesis which make up what are called "oligophrenias", even though they could probably help in our demonstration. But I am convinced that the perspective which is opened up, by stating the above is definitely worth following. To do this it is necessary and sufficient to understand what we have said on the question of the structuring and integration of a person into a reasoning being. This brings us, I realize, to the problem of the Reason, for when we speak of the personality, the self—and its world or *Dasein*—this refers us necessarily back to the dynamic structure of the individualization of the subject into a reasonable being.

As we have already noted with regard to the system of the personality, this last is built up by passing through successive phases of organization.

First, the subject starts by being *dependent on the knowledge of the objective world*. That is to say that with the opportunity that language introduces into his relationships, he learns to form his thoughts along logical lines and he integrates or incorporates into his being the techniques and principles of the communal reasoning. No one has shown better than PIAGET this noetic (i. e., intellectual) development of the reasoning "Person", or if you prefer, his "intelligence".

The self then develops in relation to a world of emotional and social values which is in the *Weltanschauung* which is right for him. The child leaves the world of his fantasies and of imaginary, prelogical, "play" reality, and builds a system of ties and beliefs which link him to other people.

The "myself" emerges from the struggle for his own identity as a sexual person who has and takes on his own vital program, which modulates basic drives into a role in keeping with the logical and historical (in the sense of life experience) structuring of his personality.

Finally, the "self" achieves a personal style of reactions, drives and behavior patterns which constitute the individual physiognomy of his *character*—these being now a "constant" of his personality.

It is obvious that this development itself is controlled and conditioned by the environment, events and situations which make up the "historicity" of the construction of self. What is less obvious—although corresponding to a reality which will be mentioned later on—is that this organization of the "Person" against his primitive, archaic and unconscious drives requires energetic and biologic conditions, as the importance of heredity shows. But let us leave aside, for the moment, this fundamental "genetic" aspect of the self to concentrate on the way its pathology presents.

The "psychopathic personality" corresponds to the first degree of anomaly of development and pathology of character. This personality type develops rigid structures more or less different from the relative plasticity of most of our own characters.

We meet, at the second degree of agenesis or unstructuring of self, all the varieties and various forms of neurotic self-organization. Essentially, it is a question in these of an infirmity marked by a spoiling of those identifying and idealistic values which, relative to others, posit the self as the creator of and not just an actor in his personage (or personality). And here is the source of the really artificial and conflicting characteristics of the neurotic self which experiences and then represses its existential malaise by using as defenses against anxiety the techniques so well described by the psychoanalytic school. Sometimes it converts its anxiety to the somatic level (hysteria), sometimes it invests the meaning into an unconsciously sought and worked out system or punishment (obsession).

At the third plateau of self-organization—that corresponding to his *Weltanschauung* or *Dasein* in as much as the self constructs links of beliefs and emotions which unite it with its world—it is the "alienated self" which designates the pathology of this particular structured level of the personality. And it is this same "alienated self" which alters, deranges or upsets the reality system in the chronic deliriums and schizophrenias. Sometimes the victim of this delirious world drives his delirium into a corner of reality (paranoia or systematized deliriums); sometimes he juxtaposes a surreality (paraphrenia) to reality; sometimes he becomes swallowed inside himself in an autistic *Eigenwelt* (BLEULER, WYRSCH).

Finally at the lowest degree of self-unstructuring we find the demented self—and this is naturally related to the preceding discussion, as the whole history and clinical progression of "intellectual" *(vesanic)* dementia leading to Dementia praecox and finally to Schizophrenia attests. This self is characterized by the most profound disorganization, which is related to its knowledge and the whole system of logical and ethical values—really its existence as a *reasonable being*. For what defines dementia is not that it is only a loss or deterioration of intelligence but that it presupposes the crumbling of all the superior structures of the personality.

If we take the problem of mental retardation, we can find in it a further demonstration of our perspective of classification. One cannot see clearly here unless the barriers which have been artificially raised between emotional activity and intelligence are dropped. Once this is accomplished, one can consider the construction and disorganization of the personality as the *Aufbau* and *Abbau* of the self, which makes itself into a system of autonomous values and, as we have stressed above, articulates at all levels its speculative and also its practical reason into the layered forms of its reasoning personality.

While still excusing myself for the rather hasty and conjectural nature of this last part of the nosographic system implied by the concept that I am developing in this paper, and while also admitting having said too much or too little, I must state that I have desired only to indicate in what new direction the whole problem of classification in mental illness could be started.

10*

Our way of seeing the problem is effectively "upsetting", for it ends up by really erasing the distinction between symptomatic and endogenous psychoses and also between "neuroses" and "dementias"—all this being contrary to all that we have learned or are learning from other sources. We are not here for the purpose of confounding everything, but on the contrary, to rediscover the natural link which ties these psychopathological problems—which are the "loss of reason" or "loss of existential equilibrium" —together.

At the end of these reflections, this attempt to classify the acute psychoses, and this project of classifying the chronic mental illnesses—on all of which I have dwelt at length in trying to point out the new and perhaps fruitful perspectives they can open up for us—I think I have shown, in any case, the following things: 1) that what we call the mental illnesses cannot be conceived of as pure and simple autonomous entities; 2) that mental illnesses are typical forms in relation to their structure and the evolution of the regressive movement which disorganizes the psyche. 3) that the structure of the psyche (field of the conscious mind on one hand and personality as regards systematic organization of the "reasonable being" on the other) furnishes us with the basic structure of all mental illnesses and also the basic principle for their classification.

V. Fourth Thesis (Etiopathogenic): The Mental Illnesses Come from Organic Processes

The discussions of psychic versus physical causality and of etiology and pathogenesis of mental illnesses are infinite. The writers in this field, usually discouraged by the inconsistencies in their own theories, finally admit that only part of mental illness comes from psychic causality (psychogenesis) or from their physical theory (organogenesis). To such a degree that they escape from this fundamental difficulty by confessing that there is indeed cause for dividing the domain of psychiatry into two sectors—that of the psychogenic afflictions and that of somatic or symptomatic problems. We, who have just established that it is necessary in clinical psychiatry to recognize a series of types which are all the result of a single unstructuring process in the psyche and whose diversity is only the result of structural differentiations of the problems of conscious mind and personality—well, we just cannot accept this idea of cutting in two the field of psychiatry. Rather we think it more correct to think of the very structure of all mental illnesses as a double complementary movement—by going back to the Jacksonian distinction between what for each one follows from its *negative structure* and *positive structure*.

1. The Distinction and Articulation of Negative and Positive

This distinction is fundamental to the very definition of the etiopatho-genic process of mental illnesses. We have previously established (in the second thesis) that a mental illness is *essentially* a regressive or inferior form of the organization of the conscious mind or personality—and this whether the illness be psychosis or neurosis, acute or chronic, or again, at a given level of psychic dissolution. This regression implies, both in its structuring and in the production of symbols, a fall into automatism, the imaginary or primitive forms of experience or of personal development. And it is this regression which represents in our eyes the *psychiatric fact* itself, a fact which offers itself to us and imposes itself on us, in all its reality, by altering the reality of experience and of the relationship of the self to its world. This idea of a deficient structure, implicit in all aspects of mental pathology is therefore the basic idea in psychiatry. No psychiatry is possible which does not comprehend the pathologic form of humanity as a structure which, by its quality of impenetrability, automatism and internal requirements escapes from the normal rules of experience and coexistence. One can term this fundamental negative structure as a "disorganization", "destructuring", "weakness of self", "agenesis", "disequilibrium", "decom-pensation". One can, even while refusing to use these terms, continue to speak of "schizophrenia", "confusion", "behavior disorder", "psychopathic personality deviations" or even "breakdown in the system of communica-tion", "change in relationship of the signifying and implied", etc.... It will be clear to whoever thinks about all this that *all* these concepts come back to the negative structure of mental illness, whether implicitly or explicitly.

Well, this *negativity* is identical with the very idea of *process*. This is quite clear if one remembers the famous theories of JASPERS. These refer to the distinction between *Verstehen* and *Erklären* which was intro-duced by DROYSEN and DILTHEY (cf. KEHRER's small book to which I have referred before). According to this way of thinking—which has become a *Leitmotiv* of contemporary psychiatric thinking—a mentally ill person cannot be analyzed by the *comprehensive* method using psychological motivation (that is, unless the illness provides something tangible which permits it to be defined). This negativity falls necessarily into the area of *explications* by the natural sciences as to the dependence of its life experience, its structural dynamism and its evolution, on a process. This process is still called a "third person process" because it is both a *factor* which limits, alters and disturbs the freedom of intersubjective relationships and also an object of the natural sciences—the "wall of biology" as FREUD once said.

The quite bizarre concept of *psychic causality* prevents mental illness from being considered as what it so obviously is. This concept usually

goes by the name *psychogenesis,* which is supposed to imply that a phenomenon which originates from this causality is related to psychic life in the
same way it would be to whatever caused it. This idea naturally demands
analysis. Just what is it supposed to mean?

It would appear that three principal aspects can be discerned in the
causality. When we say that a knock on our door is not a simple mechanical
noise but is rather the effect of some person's intention, this knock has a
meaning which links the phenomenon to an *intention,* and we therefore say
"Come in!" When we say that a child is unhappy because it has lost its
mother, we are saying that its suffering is caused by a *situation,* for this
sentiment seems to depend on a normal reservoir of events—a *motif*—and
we feel sorry for him and help him, without thinking that he is sick. And
finally, when we say that a man spent all his money because of remorse for
having illegally gained it, we are saying that his actions are caused by a
motive which we see more clearly than he himself does; we are penetrating
into the region of his emotions and tendencies just as we do all day long in
our existential relationships which are essentially intersubjective. Environ-
mental orientation, motivation and motive make up the triple meaning of
causality which drives the thought, action and language of men. It can be
added that these three modalities merge into one whole which expresses and
forms the foundation for the relationship of intersubjective understanding
which permits each and every one of us to *project* ourselves in the *direction*
of our existence.

Well, the use of this concept in mental pathology is limited by the very
structure of mental illness which we have described. And this is true even
in the case of the neuroses. Even if a given person had, in effect, the "intention" of becoming ill, this would not be sufficient to define an hysteria which
is not a conscious simulation. If this person is upset because he has lost a
loved one, his depression is not caused by the mourning but by its symbolic
and unconscious meaning with regard to the lost object. If he seeks by all
available means not to enjoy living, it is not because he wants only to be
unhappy, but because unhappiness is the unconscious goal he is pursuing.
In short, psychogenesis, in questions of mental illness, always refers us back
to the *disease causing power of the unconscious.*

This is really saying that there is a problem with unconscious drives.
But this problem cannot be thought of away from the very structure of the
psyche, which is really the organization of the conscious mind and the
personality *against* the unconscious. And this is only saying that psychic
causality—as meant and intentional causality—can be applied to mental
disease only to the degree that the psyche is so badly organized or dis-
organized that it becomes the prisoner of unconscious forces. For pure
psychic causality is viable only to the degree in which a man is normal, i. e.,

can, by his correct organization, have intentions, motifs and motives which are free from their unconscious infrastructures.

That is why the very model of mental illness is supplied by the sleep-dream phenomenon. The symbolism of dreams presents and is constituted as experience, only to the extent that it is the *prisoner* of sleep—and not only its *guardian,* as FREUD said. And this model is certainly valid for all verbal utterances, defenses, beliefs and fictional imaginings of the mentally ill. There are only two ways to break through all these phenomena and to relate them to their unconscious significance: 1) that the psychic structure be so upset that the "revived" unconscious (as in delirium or schizophrenia) reveals its secret without the sick person becoming by this act well again; 2) that the psychic structure be so little altered—as in neurosis—that the deciphering of the unconscious is made more difficult by the neurotic structuring of the self which is repressing it. But in the last analysis, in these two cases, the hermeneutic which tries to grasp the psychogenesis of the symptoms meets head on with the formal structure of the pathological existence and experiences, just as it meets the structural opacity of experience in dream analysis. All this has been discussed at length many times, but I should say with a special depth in the great discussions we had at Bonneval in 1947. And I can only refer to these ardent controversies which are, I believe, still currently of some interest.

As for me, I took a position which was quite difficult for me to take. I was steeped in psychogenesis and sociogenesis as was the whole generation of psychiatrists who were taught psychiatry as if it were a mechanism which was the only object of an extreme organicist theory, and thus I was seduced by the more dynamist and open perspectives which psychoanalysis and sociology brought in. But I quickly saw that both psychiatry and the very definition of mental illness were incompatible with this theory of psychic causality. In effect, this theory can only lead to the removal of all pathologic qualities from both neurosis and psychosis by not taking into account their *negative structure*—i. e., the basis of their pathological structure. This *negative structure* naturally isolates them—in whole or in part—from normal intentions, motifs and motives. It even, more generally, removes them from the significance which is and must be so closely *integrated* into the superior structures of the psyche if *normality* is to exist.

Finally—and here again I remember so much important thinking and work, especially that of CANGHILEM and H. MÜLLER-SUUR—mental illness is not only an abstraction but a reality, in as much as it is a qualitative deviation from the "normal type" of man. And no *meaning* can be given as the one single cause of this directional deviation.

Mental illness is then obviously a *disease (maladie)* in its deepest aspect, for it is irreducible to the very notion of psychogenesis (for one can only apply this last as a form of unconscious causality, which puts in question the force of the unconscious—i. e., the weakness of the conscious mind). And in this area, as KURT SCHNEIDER has written: "Krankheit ist immer körperlich; Krankheit gibt es nur in Leiblichen; Krankheit heißen wir seelisch abnormes Sein dann, wenn es von Krankheit verursacht ist."

Therefore we must now think of mental illness as a sickness, i. e., determined by a physical causality which limits psychogenesis, i. e., the psychic causality of the thought and action of a normal man. But just what can we make of this physical causality? It is related to the notion of a *somatic generating process*, that is, the problems, malformations, and the immaturity or disintegration which make up this causality. And certainly K. JASPERS spoke of a "psychic process" and even of "development of the personality". But it truly appears that neither schizophrenia, paranoia, nor even the neuroses can be connected to such a psychogenic causality as comes from the most thorough analysis of these disease forms. These forms always prove to be the manifestation of an upsetting or regression of the psyche and not in any way just reactions or the projection of psychic forces which normally come into play in the variations of our "relationship-filled" lives or the viscissitudes of our existence.

This said and clearly said, how can we conceive the action, development, nature, pathogenesis and "pathoplasty" (BIRNBAUM) of mental illnesses by this process? It is here that we run into JACKSON's principle concerning the articulation of negative and positive. For him the illness does not create but "liberates" ("release"). That is, it disorganizes an integrated system and initiates a reorganization at a lower level. And there is the main point, because what it really means is that the relating of a mental illness, or a manic or melancholic crisis, a schizophrenic psychosis or an hysterical neurosis to a process of malformation or disorganization does not involve the direct dependence of symptoms on "lesions". This is only admitting that the organized state falls into the inferior levels of its organization by means of a process of dissolution. And therefore we are led to acknowledge that the clinical picture does not consist of a fortuitous mosaic of non-significant symptoms, but rather represents an intentional and meaningful structure. It is precisely this concept of a generative process—so clearly shown for aphasia by JACKSON, HEAD and GOLDSTEIN—which is even more strongly valid in psychiatry. In effect, in the pathology of the conscious mind and "person" (i. e., the area of integration itself) all destructive forces do not directly lead to symptoms but only to a form of existence or *Dasein* on which symptoms depend *secondarily*. Everything takes place as if the process acted only *indirectly* and as if its effect was only of "second degree". And this is why the most monumental work of modern psychiatry—that of BLEULER on the "schizophrenic group"—stressed the double structure, both primary-negative and secondary-positive of the schizophrenic process. This famous distinction has frequently been discussed and elaborated on.

MAYER-GROSS (1930) has rightly remembered that BLEULER was thus very close to JACKSON (a comparison I systematically took up in 1947) and has pointed out that only by starting from an energetic and dynamic point of view can one then talk about a negative primary structure or process and of a positive secondary structure or psychogenesis. It is quite useless and artificial to try to make up a list of negative and positive symptoms, which prove unamenable to any distinction, to be used in practice—as has been shown in interminable discussions on this subject. If this last is true, then it is no less true that the shadow cast on the clinical picture by this process must be just as characteristic of deeper aspects of illness. In effect the *Hintergrund* or negative aspect of disease is made up of the following: this atmosphere of problems of form, the various modalities of the presentation and distribution of what is lived *(vécu)* in the pathologic experience, the qualities of incoercibility, automatism and upheaval. It is only on this base that significant forms *(Gestalten)* of the conscious mind during its pathological existence can be built, i. e., the remaining and active *positivity*.

We can point out here that in the personality disorders and in the hierarchy they form, the superior levels (schizophrenia, deliriums, neuroses) permit a great activity of pathologic production. So that the liberation *(Freisetzung)* and the compensating labors of primitive drives—(compensatory imagination, symbolic thought, uncontrolled action sequences, flood of unconscious emotions; all these being symptoms typical of what KRETSCHMER called hypoboulic and hyponoiac phenomena)—are such and the clinical picture so "florid" (JANSNIK), that a superficial observer is convinced that a pure creative *positive* force is at work. And if I have specifically stressed the importance of this positive part of the structure of mental illnesses— particularly the neuroses and psychoses of the superior level—it is because sometimes the organodynamic concept of mental illness is reproached for reducing these diseases only to a sort of negative skeleton, which is really a misinterpretation.

Thus in our perspective of things, the formation and production of symptoms requires the double dimension of both negative and positive, or more exactly their articulation, or even better still their complementary nature. These two pathogenic aspects of mental illness are nothing other than two poles or sides of the same mechanism, i. e., regression.

2. Regression as Organo-dynamic Causality—The Organo-clinical Gap

The etiopathogenic problem in mental illness sends us once again to the notion of regression (or to its twin idea, agenesis, which we will not take up here in the interest of clarity). This idea corresponds exactly to *the very function of the concept of causality as applied in the area of psychiatry*. The psychic life is either the effect of a psychogenic causality which motivates each of its actions or states of being, or else the effect, not of a physical causality pure and simple which would be meaningless, but of a proper causative force, the disorganization of a preexisting order. Certainly this application of the principle of causality is probably valid for all pathology, and I have elsewhere retraced its history. But it is much more apparent and important in the domain of psychopathology. For the life of relating, which we live out, is a hierarchical and dynamic structure whose equilibrium is naturally more precarious than that of the life force in the organism. The proper causation for mental illnesses is therefore the concept of regression or disorganization of the psyche. In other words, this causality ends up by necessarily introducing a "third person" process which upsets the unity and power of the subject (or first person). The reality of this process can only be that of a physical heterogeneity which corresponds to the very idea of a *somatogenesis*. But whether it be a question of cerebral afflictions, encephalitides, atrophies, circulatory troubles or dysmetabolic and hormonal difficulties, toxic or infectious factors, never can all these factors, as necessary as they are, be sufficient to account for the totality of the generating process. One must understand clearly that between the various mental illnesses—under whatever psychotic or neurotic aspects they show, or regarding their somatic determinism—the psychogenic action is always and necessarily interposed and is represented by the activity of the inferior levels of organization, i. e., the unconscious drives of imagination and instinct. I propose to place this divergence between the generating organic process and the clinical picture under the title *Organo-clinical Gap*, as this stresses the immanence, throughout the structure of mental illness, of an unconscious productivity which is really "endogenous".

3. Mental Illness and Central Nervous System Pathology

This same divergence or gap shows up also in the relation of the *brain* and *thought*, and consequently also in the relationship of psychiatry to the *anatomophysiologic sciences of the nervous system*. This goes back to what we have already said on the relation of neurology to psychiatry, but requires some further explanations.

Contemporary neurophysiology is essentially marked by what are called *the grand functional non-specific systems*. If, in the era of WERNICKE and HITZIG, CHARCOT and DEJERINE—i. e., the great classical period of neurology at the end of the nineteenth century—neurologists and neurophysiologists were truly obsessed by the idea of *specific functional centers*, the contemporary school of neurophysiology is going progressively away from this *idée fixe*. And PICK, HEAD, GOLDSTEIN, MONAKOW, and MOURGUE had already started matters in this direction. But the experimental research—notably in neurophysiology—which was based on the study of direct, spontaneous, provoked or evoked electrical potentials was decisive in this regard. These innumerable papers—the work of MAGOUN, MORUZZI, LORENTE DE NO, BREMER, H. H. JASPER, GASTAUT, etc., or the experimental data from "acute preparations" and the psychobiology of "chronic preparations", or even the discoveries of neurochemistry and the microphysiology of synapses—all this work ended by giving validity to the concept of "non-specific functional centers". The profound interest of our knowledge of the great ascending reticular system (AARS) articulated with the reticulo-bulbar (both ascending and descending) and thalamic inhibitory systems—this last in regard to the tone of alertness—is well known. Great importance has thus been attached to this old brain or "centrencephalon" (PENFIELD) both by the anatomophysiologic connections of this longitudinal and axial system with the limbic lobe, and by the role of all the meso-diencephalo-rhinencephalic formations in the instinctive-emotional activities of the brain (the Los Angeles school—KAADA, MACLEAN, OLDS, etc.). I have myself (Tome III of the *Etudes*) tried to show that the pathology of these encephalic formations was structurally tied not only to the function of vigilance-alertness, but also to the pathology of the field of the conscious mind. It is quite possible that the future—already foreshadowed by the papers of the cyberneticians (GRAY WALTER, W. ASHBY, N. WIENER, MAC CULLOCH, etc.) or the work of SCHOLL, LASHLEY, HEBB, etc.—will see new progress achieved in our empirical and speculative knowledge of structure as "feedback", the reverberations of information and the significant reservoir of "probability" of nervous activity. Everything seems to take place as if the brain were not only the *seat* of functional centers but also the *agent* of a system of functional relationships having its own energies. Even though these various intuitions are still vague and premature, it is no less true that the relationship of psychiatry and the brain must pass more naturally through this type of synergically functioning brain than through the centers of projection and association of Fleching of one hundred years ago. The famous Anglo-Saxon "Symposia" on this theme are of great interest— London Symposium of 1950, Ste. Marguerite, 1954, Ciba Foundation, 1957, and that directed and edited by H. D. KRUSE in 1957 on *Integrality— The Approach to Mental Diseases*. It will suffice just to think of these symposia in order to reflect on the conceptual and experimental difficulties of this highly functional aspect of the central nervous system.

In this perspective, the *cerebral gray matter* would appear to be the organ of functional differentiation or Gestaltization necessary for the "analyses" (the ideas of a perceptual analyzer and of the second conditioning system of PAVLOV), filtering, and reading out of messages, signals and information. Although we were thrown off momentarily by the concept of hegemony of the reticular system of the brainstem, it did not take us long to see that this system of analysis and elaboration is itself articulated (or hooked into) the specific, energetic and functional centers, forming with them a vast system of cortical-reticular rebound or reverberation.

In this functional unity of the integration of psychic life, one can and must discern two possibilities for disintegration: 1) the instrumental disorganization of relatively isolable functions (-gnosias, -praxias, a system of verbal expressions, perceptions, etc.) which make up the traditional concerns of neurology, and 2) the unstructuring of the grand organizational forms of the psyche which are the natural concern of psychiatry. According to LLAVERO, psychiatry cannot be "anencephalic" and we also must necessarily articulate our structural and phenomenological analyses with the very organization of the brain. Which organization is not, to use the famous witticism of R. W. GERARD, the celebrated neurologist: "a ball of string wound up in the skull" *(un paquet de cordon cardé dans le crâne),* but is rather an ensemble of vital structuring, a marvelous work of morphology, as K. JASPERS said. And the whole problem—which is at the very heart of our organodynamic concept, at least as an axis of orientation for research and progress—is, on one hand, in the *articulation* of the structure and unstructuring of the psyche, and on the other hand, in the organization and disorganization of the brain. In this regard, the retreat of the specific functional center in the face of the newly elaborated cerebral energetic "patterns" seems to have started the problem in a new and fruitful direction for research, whose program enters quite naturally into our hypothesis.

But it is clear that in this new perspective, mental problems, while depending on cerebral pathology, should not be mixed up purely and simply with the "determinant" and conditioning of this pathology. The organization of the nervous system is not that of the psyche, but is only the accessory condition for it, which leaves in psychic activity enough play or freedom for it to achieve relative autonomy. It is here that our hypothesis moves away from that inspired by a monistic mechanism which would appear indefensible to us. For between the brain and actual behavior lies the "atopical" organization of the value system, which constitutes personality. Thus the unstructuring of the psyche, while coming out of its negative form of cerebral disorganization, depends also and necessarily on the workings or proper dynamics of psychic activity.

4. The Exotoxic Processes

This multidimensional aspect (KRETSCHMER, BIRNBAUM) of the structure of mental illness is particularly evident in the toxic processes. These are at present making news—a fact which would make MOREAU DE TOURS, KRAEPLIN, BUMKE, REGIS, etc., smile (and these are only the great classical names). Certainly it is not a question here of a recent psychopathological discovery since all the great clinicians, and FREUD himself, have always considered that the study of nervous system poisons and intoxicants is of central interest for psychiatry. But what can be considered as a truly new contribution is the sheer number of pharmacological agents at present, and their particularly psychotropic qualities, for which they are so widely used in psychopharmacology and in the provoking of "model psychoses". Having said this, it is no less true that the study of the unstructuring of the conscious mind, which these psychotropic substances provoke, shows merely that they are acting on a functional edifice, or rather on a dynamic and hierarchical structure of the psyche—in that they do not provoke truly "mechanical" symptoms but rather regressions which are the result of the negative and positive factors which are brought to bear. And it is in this way that these states of intoxication constitute a sort of experimental model for the mental illnesses.

5. Heredo-degenerative Processes

But no process can be envisaged only in its exogenous form, for especially as regards the pathology of the personality (i. e., which means most of the endogenous psychoses), the heredo-genetic factors play an extremely important role. *The hereditary aspect of mental illness is a fact of supreme importance.* And it is not sufficient to employ "la politique de l'autriche" to erase this fact, as do the psychoanalysts, sociopsychiatrists, etc.; even as one cannot reduce it to an overly strict and artificial Weismanian or Mendelian interpretation. This fact is there in front of us, as if to remind us constantly that, the problem of madness being immanent in human nature, malformations of the psyche are serious predisposing conditions. But I repeat, it is not a question of trying once again to use the indefensible distinction of symptomatic vs. endogenous to distinguish between disease of the conscious mind and that of the personality. For heredity and exogenous factors collaborate in the determining and etiopathogenic production of all and any generatory processes. I have desired simply to stress here *in fine* that when sceptical minds demand what proof we have of the organicity of the determinism of the neuroses, schizophrenias or paranoias, it is the empirical study of hereditary risks, inheritance and consanguinity of these illnesses which will reply to them (cf. my report on "l'Hérédité des Maladies Mentales" in *Journées de Bonneval*, 1950, and my more recent article on "l'Hérédité des Nevroses", *Evolution Psychiatrique*, 1959).

Finally, let us say just how I have established, in the case of the schizophrenic process, that the somatic process is confused with the tendencies of the personality, with the object, the degree of disorganization and the evolutionary potential of mental illnesses. For the process of regression is at the same time a condition of impotence (negative structure) and a need (positive structure). Such is the double, functionally coordinated way in which the movement toward disorganization in the psyche is registered in all forms and at all levels.

VI. Practical Corollaries

In closing let us try to say something about the practical value of the working hypothesis whose essential theoretical positions we have just elaborated, in all their ramifications.

1. The Distinction between Normal and Pathological

The organodynamic concept of mental pathology gives major importance to the structural differences between *normal* and *pathological* in all areas (cultural, medicolegal, religious, esthetic) for this distinction is fundamental to psychiatry. It also fills a need which is of great practical importance. In effect it is not sufficient to say—as is so often reiterated—that all men are mad, which is like saying that no one really is. If madness is immanent in and pervades the structure of the psyche which contains it, it is created only by the effect of a regressive process which gives a formal character to the symptomatology. From then on if, in fact, it is difficult to make a diagnosis, there is at least, by all rights, a basis for one. And this is at least a step forward relative to so many "bastard" concepts which remain, with regard to this problem of first rank, indifferent or impotent as to its formulation or the practical consequences following from it.

Naturally it is in the area of spiritual and moral values and with the problem of penal responsibility and civilian capacity that the psychiatrist needs to be able to lean on a psychiatric theory which supports rather than undermines his actions, methods of therapy and expertise.

From among the numerous practical applications of the discrimination between the normal and the pathological we will mention only two which have a particular importance with reference to human values.

In the area of *religious psychology*, the distinction between normal and pathologic turns up in a dramatically demanding fashion. I have encountered several times the very difficult problems related to religious vocations, the value of mystical experiences and also the morbid character of guilt and self-accusation. And always my purpose was to show that if, in fact, the discussion of a diagnosis is sometimes embarrassing, the clinical studying of the pathologic, when it is well done, can and must save us from this fearful embarrassment.

As for *psychopathological art,* I have also shown that only in depth analyses can posit (ask) and resolve the problem of values:

There it's a question of a "cream pastry" for all those psychiatrists who are not well informed in literature or artistic erudition. So much so that well done studies on this theme are rare (relative to the fantastic number of articles published, especially on painting—BOSCH, VAN GOGH, the Expressionists, the Surrealists, etc.). I have *(Evolution Psychiatrique,* 1938) tried to break with this obsolete tradition—which unceasingly renews itself—which consists of comparing the works of artists with those of the sick. All reflections on such comparisons only end up by repeating the premise from which they began: i. e., that the fantastic or poetic are *analogous* in either group to the expression of the unconscious. I have tried to show that the problem doesn't lie in this *analogy* but in analysis of why these things were produced. And it is in this regard that there is such a great difference between *making* a work of art and *being* oneself fantastic and marvelous. But I fear that all hope has come to naught of introducing into this question the necessity of a structural and phenomenological analysis to emphasize its differential nature and not just make an analogous comparison.

2. Reconsideration of Nosographic Problems

Our hypothesis also permits the opening of *new perspectives in clinical psychiatry.* The job of observation and classification of disease types is far from being outmoded or finished. Clinical psychiatry is on the contrary engaged in fruitful clinical studies indispensable for the drawing up of rules of diagnosis and prognosis of the mental illnesses which unstructure the field of the conscious mind and also those which disorganize the system of the personality. By abandoning a certain number of artificial distinctions (for example that of the endogenous vs. exogenous psychoses) and by retaining the most valuable clinical analyses of our predecessors, we have before us a vast field of action. But only, in conformity with our hypothesis, if we reject also the notion of entities plus the idea that there are no structural types of mental illnesses.

3. The Necessity for a Symptomatology of the Depths of the Psyche

This theoretical position permits the integration of the *Tiefenpsycho-logie* and especially the *discoveries* of FREUD and the psychoanalytic school into the clinical approach. This position also orients our clinical studies in the direction of the penetration and deciphering of the symbols lived and experienced by the man who becomes the prisoner of his fantasies. But it avoids falling into the excess of a hermeneutic "at any cost". Said another way, it achieves a point of equilibrium between form and content and negative and positive which is precisely the point of contact between psycho-analysis and psychiatry and also between existential and clinical analysis.

4. Neuro-physiologic Perspectives

The organodynamic concept of psychiatry, far from excluding and instead demanding its new knowledge of somatic determinism (cerebral, neurophysiological, hormonal, etc.), backs up the validity of the neurologic and biologic research in psychiatry and is launching them toward a concept of cerebral energy which superimposes itself on the functions and localizations of the brain.

5. Therapeutic Perspectives

In therapeutic activity, the hypothesis that we have been discussing accounts at the same time for the efficacity and limits of psychotherapy, and in a more general way implies a convergence of biological and psychotherapeutic methods of treatment. In this regard, if it is true that (as we are assured in *The Life and Times of Sigmund Freud*, E. JONES, 1953, page 259) FREUD was convinced that one day drugs would do more than psychotherapy; and if he established that chemotherapy has made and will make still greater progress, we can only say that the dynamo-organic concept expressed and foresaw all this. But there again, by its very hypothesis, it admits that no pure psychotherapy (except by ignorance of the spontaneous movement in the evolving illness) and no exclusively chemical or biological method of treatment (other than by misunderstanding the other psychological aspects of its action) can totally and definitely cure a mentally ill person who is at the same time an organically malformed and altered patient, and also a man who is living out a drama that only the aid of another person can help him overcome.

6. Helpful Suggestions

Finally, concerning all the theoretical and practical problems (help, organization of services and professions) raised by the relationship of psychiatry with medicine and especially neurology, the organodynamic theory of mental illnesses integrates psychiatry into medicine while still radically distinguishing and separating it from organ pathology. The rapports with neurology are of the same type. For psychiatry is separate in this regard in that it is a pathology, not of the vitality or key functions of a life of relatedness, but rather a pathology of humanity, liberty and existence.

Thus we are touching with our finger—at the end of this overly long (or too brief) discussion—the exact meaning of the organodynamic concept of psychiatry. Its purpose is to be a *Natural History of Madness*. "History" as anthropological science of the *subject*, decapitated, as it were, of the human values which make up his historicity. "Natural history" as a natural science whose *concern* is the process of regression which disorganizes the organism and therefore the psyche which comes from it.

As an *organodynamic* theory it constitutes a hypothetical interpretation of mental diseases which are thus defined as organic constructions of the disorganization (organic process) which creates them. To be mentally ill is therefore for a man to fall under the influence of the determinism of his organism. In this respect, this theory assumes a psychodynamic theory of normal psychology. One can now comprehend, in its fundamental nature, the misinterpretation of those psychodynamic concepts being applied to an object—mental illness—which is radically inadequate for their particular theory.

And so we have the final word on this concept of which each person must judge if it is only a pure a priori construction or a simple eclectic juxtaposition of contradictory ideas; in short, if it is nothing—or if it really reaches into the very reality of the structure and disorganization of psychic life. Perhaps the very coherence of the theses which make it up is a guarantee—if not proof—of its validity.

Bibliography

EY (Henri) et ROUART (Julien): Essai d'application des principes de Jackson à une conception dynamique de la Neuro-Psychiatrie. *Encéphale* 1936.

EY (Henri): Etudes psychiatriques (3 volumes). Paris: Ed. Desclée de Brouwer. Tome I: Historique, méthodologie, psychopathologie générale. 1ère édition 1948, 296 p. — 2ème édition revue et augmentée, 1952. Tome II: Aspects séméiologiques. 1ère édition 1950, 547 p. — 2ème édition, 1957, sans modification. Tome III: Structure des psychoses aiguës et déstructuration de la conscience. 1ère édition 1954, 787 p. — 2ème édition 1960, sans modification.

— Encyclopédie Médico-Chirurgicale (Psychiatrie), Paris 1955. Sous la direction de HENRI EY avec 132 collaborateurs, 3 volumes in-quarto. Ed. Encyclopédie Médico-Chirurgicale, 18 rue Séguier, Paris VIème.

— La conscience. 1ère édition, P. U. F., Paris 1963, 439 p. — 2ème édition, P. U. F., Paris 1968, 500 p.

— Le phénomène sommeil-rêve dans ses rapports avec la psychopathologie. (Théorie de la relativité généralisée et de l'Etre conscient en Psychiatrie.) IV World Congress of Psychiatry, Madrid 1966. Amsterdam: Ed. Excerpta Medica Foundation 1968.

Typesetting and printing: Konrad Triltsch, Graphischer Betrieb, Würzburg

DATE DUE

MAY 1 1979			
1 1990			